MENTAL HEALTH PROMOTION

MENTAL HEALTH PROMOTION

Policy, Practice and Partnerships

Gary F McCulloch
BA (Hons), RMN, Dip HP
Senior Health Promotion Specialist – Mental Health, Sheffield Health,
Sheffield, UK

Judy Boxer
RMN, CQSW, RNT
Formerly Nurse Lecturer, School of Nursing, Faculty of Medicine,
University of Sheffield, Sheffield, UK

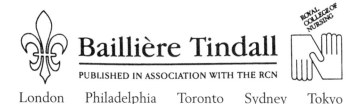

Baillière Tindall
PUBLISHED IN ASSOCIATION WITH THE RCN

London   Philadelphia   Toronto   Sydney   Tokyo

Baillière Tindall   24–28 Oval Road
London NW1 7DX

The Curtis Center
Independence Square West
Philadelphia, PA 19106-3399, USA

Harcourt Brace & Company
55 Horner Avenue
Toronto, Ontario, M8Z 4X6, Canada

Harcourt Brace & Company, Australia
30–52 Smidmore Street
Marrickville
NSW 2204, Australia

Harcourt Brace & Company, Japan
Ichibancho Central Building
22-1 Ichibancho
Chiyoda-ku, Tokyo 102, Japan

A catalogue record for this book is available from the British Library

ISBN 0-7020-1981-X

Typeset by Poole Typesetting (Wessex) Limited
Printed and bound in Great Britain by Bath Press, Bath

Contents

Introduction

The invention of madness as a disease is in fact nothing less than a peculiar disease of our civilization. We choose to conjure up this disease in order to evade a certain moment of our own existence – the moment of disturbance, of penetrating vision into the depths of ourselves, that we prefer to externalize into others. Others are elected to live out this chaos that we refuse to confront in ourselves. By this means we escape a certain anxiety, but only at a price that is as immense as it is unrecognised.
(Cooper 1971)

Overview

In this text we will highlight and address the most salient issues in relation to mental health and its promotion. We will place in context and argue for the importance of mental health promotion (MHP) in its own right. To do this we need to distinguish between mental health education and promotion, and consider why MHP is something that requires working towards and supporting. It is not necessarily something that practitioners will perceive and do something about as part of their core activity. On the contrary, the assumption that MHP is embedded within the training, practice and philosophy of health and social care, is just that – an assumption.

Introduction

We write this book at a time of immense change and upheaval. The crisis in health and social welfare continues and the future of our welfare needs is high on the agenda of the Labour Government. The growth and investment in the private and voluntary sectors in propping up the previous Conservative government's economic vision continues to have a major impact on the lives of individuals and the communities in which they live and work. The change in emphasis from institution-alized care to locally-based services is underfunded and piecemeal, with professionals seemingly ill-equipped to cope with the conflictual nature of mental illness and how this 'problem' should be addressed within a comprehensive framework of health and social care. At the same time as more and more people are being cared for in the community, there is an underlying message that it is still the order of the day to lock people up, even if the failure is in the circumstance or the policy, not the individual. Hence the massive increase in the prison population, in secure psychiatric provision, and in the 'mini' institutions springing up, especially in the private sector, which still mirror the problem of institutionalized living. Increasingly, there has been a realization that unless the values which underpin decent human existence and cooperation are re-examined and instilled in people in a more positive way, our society is in danger of fragmenting further.

This has major implications for our mental health, however much this is skirted over by politicians and the 'moral majority'. It is easy to remain negative and pessimistic. The task is an impossible one. Someone else will sort out the mess we have got ourselves into. The age-old arguments about absolute and relative poverty and the relationship to ill-health and mental health problems still rage as more people become disenfranchised from a meaningful existence, even if they can fill in their lottery tickets every week. The numbers of people experiencing or living in conditions which constitute 'poverty' cannot be denied, yet we know that when people become disadvantaged they have little power or voice to be heard. The philosophy of individualism pervades all aspects of our lives in some vain attempt to attain the 'freedom' that most of us would not know what to do with if we had it. The main focus of this book is about the 'freedoms' which relate to our emotional well-being and opportunities for personal growth and development. That this is still inextricably linked to our basic identity is a sad reflection on how little importance we place on individual worth and how so many people can be disadvantaged in this process. The high incidence of abuse, rape, domestic violence and neglect of our children in this country, if not in all parts of the world, is also an indication of the onus of responsibility placed on the individual, usually within a sanctioned existence such as the family, to cope with untenable relationships and circumstances. The relationships between individuals, the professionals who are supposed to support those in this position, and the state's investment in achieving cohesion in society, collide head on when one group of people is deemed 'insane' and another not. The theoretical vision that spans these concerns, from moral philosophy to psychoanalytic to postmodern accounts of individual and social existence, cannot be explored in any real depth in our account, however much these subjects interest us and have informed our thinking.

As a concept, mental health promotion is relatively new. The advantage of this is that it provides an opportunity to think creatively within a social framework of health. The downside is that limited theoretical debate can result in it being seen as all things to all people. This dilemma has to be recognized by all concerned, and the reasons why this might be the case. What we do recognize is a climate of increasing awareness of emotional health and a cultural shift towards health as positive well-being. Our environment and economic and social structures are increasingly being seen in relation to quality of life. Unfortunately, in staking a claim for positive mental health the agendas of the public, professionals, and the state conflict on many levels, especially in terms of ideology and economic investment. In this book we allude to the need for greater consideration of what constitutes 'ethical practice', and debates about justice and care need to be given a much higher profile in how we 'promote' mental health in the context of the world we live in.

For us, MHP concerns the fundamentals of mental health and is inextricably linked to our general health and social welfare. It could be accused of not being at the sharp end of severe mental illness. However, even the most hardened traditionalists who work within the medical model do not see psychopharmocology and 'treatment' as the sole solution to mental ill-health in acute or enduring presentations. It is acknowledged that we all have mental health needs and that they cannot so easily be distanced from our physical health, or that holistic interpretation can more realistically inform who we are as individuals, within a complex and changing environment. Our interpersonal and social world, our values, and economic and learning potential all inter-relate and need addressing. While these may not be the sole preserve of the medical or nursing professions, whose main activity is to treat and to care, the process by which this is achieved is in the formation and sustaining of social relationships. However manufactured such relation-ships may be, they are essential for the management and treatment of mental illness and are deemed vital for our emotional well-being if we do not have the capacity to make these choices ourselves. The central-ity of such relationships to mental illness service provision is considered as one of the problem areas and any reading of the history of psychiatry and mental health practice provides a depressing account of the failures of 'therapeutic intervention'. It is no coincidence that the emphasis on psychotherapeutic/counselling approaches and alternative therapies has a much higher profile these days, and that these approaches are increas-ingly informing mainstream practice to counteract these deficiencies.

We are all in some ways mental health 'experts'. In our relatively 'unconscious' use of verbal and nonverbal communication, the over-whelming majority of us are fluent and sophisticated in forming and developing relationships and ideas and acting upon them in a range of ways. Sympathy, empathy and support for others and our own need for this make mental health the most individual and collective of experiences. This is nurtured or hindered by love, envy, power, greed, control, autonomy, freedom and opportunity for emotional growth. Our mental and emotional state is central to our life and style of life. We also have an experience and appreciation of our own and others' emotional health. We sense when things are not right and we are pretty clear when it comes to someone being so emotionally distressed that they require more than we can offer. This is as important for our own well-being as it is for that of our fellow citizens. Why some people survive and others do not is probably one of the unanswerables, but the boundaries to this are obviously blurred by history, economy and power. We tend to know where we stand, if not quite knowing why.

Our mental health relates to our 'consciousness' of the subjective, emotional elements that distinguish us from other creatures. Given the right circumstances we experience a quality of life which is significant and worthwhile. Without these we are emotionally starved and can quickly become mentally unwell. This inevitably leads people down the slippery slope to mental illness, and its consequent 'treatment' by professionals. It is an important area, emotional in itself, and one in which degrees of prevention and elements of education to demystify the reality of its manifestation are desirable. So too, are the emotional – the mental health – needs of the mentally ill a worthy area for action. However, the focus of our discussion will be on how we can promote and sustain mental health for *all* citizens. Doing this means promoting mental health.

If, as we intend to, we see health promotion from a Health for All framework, it is no coincidence that our travels around general population approaches to improving mental health will also include the themes of vulnerable groups, including the mentally ill. The examples and approach taken will include promoting mental health for the general population, with specific groups and within mental illness and related settings.

MHP could cynically be described as the process of getting rid of the 'ism's' – racism, sexism, ageism, medicalism – or at least considering further how they become embedded in a range of responses to our mental health needs, from attitudes to structures, systems and activities. The scope and vision of a role for mental health promotion within mainstream practice has to be very broad based and experienced as a developmental process, rather than as an academic exercise. These issues are what an 'honest' psychiatry should be addressing, but at the present time the pendulum is swinging more and more in the direction of 'scientific' credibility rather than common sense. Mental health promotion and social justice have been described as two sides of the same coin, and it is up to all of us to find ways of ameliorating the health–social care divide (Monach and Spriggs 1995).

A note on language

'But "glory" doesn't mean "a nice knock down argument"',
Alice objected.
'When I use a word,' Humpty Dumpty said in a rather scornful tone, 'it means just what I choose it to mean – neither more nor less.'
'The question is', said Alice, 'whether you can make words mean different things.'
'The question is', said Humpty Dumpty, 'which is to be master – that's all.'
(*Through the Looking Glass*, Lewis Carroll)

Throughout this text a range of phrases and definitions are used in relation to people who are or have been in contact with mental health services, particular communities and communities of interest. As Read and Wallcraft (1995) highlight, 'service user' is a problematic label, particularly for people under an element of the Mental Health Act. They also point out that some individuals who have been at the receiving end of psychiatry and its services may find terminology such as 'mental illness' oppressive in itself. With this in mind we employ the following phrases and terms throughout the text:

- Patient
- Recipient
- Client
- Service user
- User
- Survivor
- People
- Citizen

These are employed in the context of how individuals and communities of interest define themselves. We accept that such terms can be misleading, cumbersome or offensive to some people. We also refrain from such terms as 'schizophrenic', 'neurotic' and 'psychotic', and instead refer to 'people with a diagnosis of . . . ' or 'people who refer to themselves as . . . '. This latter point is important for a more sophisticated discussion. In our attempts to appreciate and respond positively to the negative power of language we can assume that people with labels may wish to discard them. On the contrary an individual or group may see a label of 'schizophrenic' or 'mad' as testimony to an identity which may have been shaped by a range of psychiatric experience. Just as, for example, black culture and gay culture have reclaimed words such as 'nigger' and 'queer', so too have some individuals and groups highlighted their sense of history and common experience by referring to themselves as 'service recipients' and 'schizophrenics'. This lexicon of the oppressed needs to be acknowledged and accepted no matter how uncomfortable it makes us feel.

In terms of the impact of language it must also be accepted, at the pragmatic level, that labels act as gatekeepers to a range of services and support. To be 'disabled' by a mental illness is to have certain rights to welfare and services available from professional agencies. The rules, regulations and paperwork allow little room for preference or political statement. However, even within the confines of information gathering and diagnostic coding, there should be opportunities for people who are in touch with services to determine for themselves, or for the record (literally and metaphorically) what they see as their human condition. We also use words and phrases in the context of how government and professional documents are presented. For example, the Butterworth Report refers to people who are receiving mental health services as 'clients' throughout the report, and we use that term in discussing its contents.

We acknowledge that there is no universal term acceptable to everyone, and that people have a range of experiences and circumstances which are difficult, if not impossible, to encapsulate under such artificial homogeneous labels as 'patient' or 'survivor'. It may be that people are all or none of these things, or have experienced some of them. A common term we employ is that of the *citizen*. This is for the political as well as the relatively neutral value such a word contains. It implies the individual but also the social individual. With citizenship come rights and responsibilities. As such we should all be party to the same rules, regulations and, equally importantly, the same justice and potential for reaching and maintaining positive mental health within a 'democratic' society.

Themes

Throughout this text we will also examine MHP in terms of practice and interventions which can shed light on how specialist and nonspecialist mental health practitioners may best develop work in this area. We also hope this book will be of value to a wide range of people, including service users. The following aspects are considered central.

Health for all

The key principles of equity, participation and collaboration will be referred to and drawn upon throughout the text. It is recognized that the pragmatic reality of work in the health service, and sadly, around mental illness and mental health all too easily papers over the social determinants of health, or they remain an annoying background hum! Part of the role of a health for all framework and a mental health-promoting approach is to raise this profile in a more comprehensive way. Bringing this to the foreground of consciousness in the domain of mental health enables practice to become something more than good professional services with health promotion added on. The added value is not only in the understanding. It is in the journey to that under-standing and recognition that the mental health professional plays a part but is perhaps not the determining factor.

Psycho-socio-cultural perspectives

An exploration of material on class, gender, age, race, ethnicity, disabil-ity, the family and the environment is necessary to support the approach we take. The text will allow the reader to evaluate the impact of bias in these areas on people's mental health and service provision and alternative approaches.

Socio-political-economic issues

What are the socio-political-economic aspects of mental health? This question involves an overview of current social policy and analysis of how such policy is impacting on mental health service provision (and planning). Issues such as equal opportunities and anti-oppressive prac-tice will also be discussed in the text to enable the reader to consider this in their own health setting.

Research and good practice

What are the key pieces of research and key research questions in rela-tion to health promotion and mental health? What developments are taking place which identify MHP as a 'concept' in its own right? The text will enable the reader to understand and critically evaluate reports and good practice approaches. This includes local health profiles, skill surveys and good practice audit.

Education and training

This is a vast subject area and obviously considers the importance of education throughout our lifetime in addressing how our mental health needs are best met. This will be dependent on economic and practical considerations, such as with the current debates within educational circles about the value of traditional education and vocational experience. Learning from life experience is probably as important as reading from any course book within this domain, and we identify the change taking place in terms of user involvement at all levels of mental health practice and provision.

Action

How can health professionals use their roles creatively to effect change at the individual, interpersonal and collective levels? What degree of reciprocation in terms of autonomy and therefore responsibility and accountability does this require? The notion of risk taking needs to be considered in relation to professionals attempting to act as advocate or lobbying for change, especially with the changes to mental health legislation currently taking place or being considered, and keeping their job.

Approach

Questions to consider

The text will frequently pose questions for reflection, discussion and debate. This will encourage the reader to question the content and formulate ideas in relation to their own practice and experience. Most chapters end with a Practice Checklist to help readers consider how they can address priorities in their own practice.

Outline of chapters

General themes

- What constitutes 'good' mental health?
- What is the national/European/international perspective?
- What are the implications of MHP for practitioners?
- How can we best evaluate strategic approaches and incorporate them into service delivery?
- How can our vision of MHP survive the journey from policy to practice?
- What implications are there for the purchasing agenda?
- How can users of services be more involved?
- Whose responsibility is it to coordinate action planning for MHP at local level?
- Is there scope for a different approach to education and training?
- What are the arguments for and against generic versus specialist workers in current mental health practice?

These aspects will be developed more specifically in each of the following chapters.

Chapter 1 sets out some of the debate and theory around mental health and illness and MHP and considers a framework for practice which will be highlighted in this chapter; in subsequent chapters these themes are put into context. Chapter 2 examines some of the key policies which inform practice and resource allocation. Given the complex nature of health and social policy level, it will focus on mental illness services but will also broaden the debate to a Healthy Cities approach and the potential role of the public health nurse. Chapter 3 establishes the importance of health alliances and community participation for MHP. Chapter 4 develops this further to look at the strategic approach and strategies relating to mental illness and mental health in practice as well developing a MHP strategic framework. Chapter 5 reveals the relationship between education and training in the mental health field and the implications for MHP work. Chapter 6 looks at prevention. The debate and research around prevention strategies are discussed and a range of action and outcomes for practitioner are identified. This includes the relevance of education within a HP framework – its limitations and potential – and realization of a way forward for practice. Chapter 7 examines current purchasing issues in terms of assessment of health needs and the role of the practitioner and the public in influencing the purchasing process for mental health. Chapter 8 has as its focus, user and carer issues; it explores the key issues and concerns from the user and carer perspective and details examples of good practice which the practitioner can tap into. Chapter 9 pulls together the main themes and proposes a way forward for MHP in practice. Chapter 10 provides a 'toolbox' of resources, activity and further examples of practice which can be used to develop MHP in community and specialist mental illness settings.

Listed at the start of each chapter are Key Themes which indicate the content and development ideas we consider most relevant. Where it has been possible, we have provided examples of policy, practice and the strategies which have been considered in relation to this subject. Suggested reading is included in Chapter 10 which supports the theoretical perspectives outlined in the relevant chapters. This is not a definitive list and there are many books which address the topics raised and consider them more specifically in terms of our physical, psychological and social needs and wants. We hope this book will provide some basis for the educational requirements of both health and social care courses, and we have included exercises and areas of discussion, debate and research. We have included a short glossary which supports the developments we consider in Chapter 5 about anti-oppressive practice, and a more radical approach to education and practice. Overall, we hope that the book is comprehensive enough for individuals to take from it what they need, whether this is further understanding of what constitutes the purchaser/provider divide, or more abstract considerations of why we approach mental illness in the way we do and what is wrong with the present 'system'.

Thanks and acknowledgements

There are many people we would wish to thank for their help, support, understanding and patience while we experienced mental health problems writing this book! This book would not have been possible without the encouragement and sound advice we received from Jacqueline Curthoys, Senior Editor at Baillière Tindall and to her we are gratefully indebted.

Mostly we feel indebted to the many people whom we have cared for, nursed and supported in very difficult and oppressive circumstances that years of working in mental health practice have revealed. The courage, warmth, generosity and openness of individuals stands out in our minds, as does being 'licked into shape' when our professional role collided with what we, or others, truly believed as human beings. Our world could fall apart just as easily, and if it did would we like to be 'treated' in the way that much of statutory provision deems acceptable?

We would also like to thank those people, both alive and those who are unfortunately no longer with us, who have given us inspiration to keep on writing and who have contributed so much to our theoretical understanding and in enhancing a more comprehensive framework for 'authentic' practice.

On a more individual note we each have family, friends and colleagues we would like to acknowledge for their love and friendship in supporting us in what at times became a very isolating, but rewarding learning process. The list would be very long, and we have decided not to mention individuals by name; they know who they are.

A framework for practice

1

Just as hysteria was a by-product of Victorian prudishness and repression, so anorexia nervosa and narcissistic personality disorder express the self-centeredness and concern with external experiences of our time. (Brizer 1993)

Key themes:

- Why mental health and health promotion?
- A model for health
- Development of a definition for MHP
- Community
- Elements for framework for MHP
- Framework
- Questions/discussion points

Overview

This chapter sets out the context for more detailed discussion of policy, strategy and practice in the area of mental health promotion. It examines a range of definitions and proposes a framework for practitioners in the field of mental health promotion. Underpinning such a framework is the necessity for anti-oppressive practice and a social model of health. There are very few books which address mental health promotion specifically, and the development of anti-oppressive practice within nursing has not been incorporated, as it has within social work education. We hope to redress that imbalance in this text, and are continuing to develop and refine our ideas in the light of recent work in this field.

Why mental health?

Mental health is important not just for its own sake but because of the meanings and actions attached to it, whether they are society's, communities', or our own. There are also considerable pressures brought to bear on us to respond and react in 'emotionally acceptable' ways. The taboo of individual and societal disruption manifest in mental illness is a reminder of shared core fears and concerns inhabiting minds and history.

Mental health is both objective and subjective: the former in terms of the neurological and biochemical–molecular foundations for thoughts and actions as well as the potential for cognition and perception of our world. The subjective, as alluded to in the introduction, relates to our understanding of being conscious, our interpretation, responses and meanings attached to the perceived world in terms of our values, ideas, emotions and their expression. The attempt to distinguish between these is usually defined as distinctions of nurture versus nature. A 'nurture' version of mental health can be said to emphasize the evolutionary, ecological and environmental factors which interact both to influence and enhance or to inhibit mental health. A 'natural' definition of mental health, on the other hand, places more emphasis on inherited disposition, of personality, behavioural responses and chemical balance or imbalance. There is no observable dividing line between subjective and objective reality, and the premise on which our ideas rest is that it is not as easy as 'scientific thinking' tells us, that the root of personal distress is categorization of mental illness.

The rationale for mental health promotion that we discuss rests clearly within a subjective view of the world. Ideologically and philosophically, a social model of health, as proposed by health promotion, makes such a distinction inevitable. As we have already considered, this does not, and should not, rule out the role of mental health promotion in the field of mental illness. Indeed, this appears to be the root of current health policy. A blend of promotion and prevention is advocated as part of Health of the Nation (DOH 1992a, 1994a). Despite the potential confusion that this may cause, it allows the three elements of health promotion to be considered and a framework for education, prevention and protection to be developed. At a pragmatic level this inevitably results in considerable discussion of mental health as it relates to mental illness.

Our mental health is the most personal, individual, private and yet the most public. Our conscious world is constantly scrutinized, interpreted, and interacted with via the social lives we lead. Our emotions, moods, views and opinions, values, thoughts, reflections and actions are all part of our mental health. Mental health is in turn influenced by these factors in others' behaviours and actions incrementally over a lifetime. We have highlighted the complexity of mental health and how difficult it therefore is to find an adequate definition. We highlight a recent definition which seems to capture the 'essence' of what mental health includes (Box 1.1). This will obviously be dependent on the variables that gender, culture, ethnicity, class, disability, age and sexuality bring to any notion of 'normality'.

Box 1.1 **Core elements of mental health**

Mental health includes the following capacities

- The ability to develop psychologically, emotionally, intellectually and spiritually
- The ability to initiate, develop and sustain mutually satisfying personal relationships
- The ability to become aware of others and to empathize with them
- The ability to use psychological distress as a development process, so that it does not hinder or impair further development

Together We Stand: Child & Adolescent Mental Health Services (DOH 1995a)

In our teaching of mental health we have undertaken many exercises to help students and practitioners explore this very personal subject. As with the development of anti-oppressive practice, care needs to be taken that people are given the right circumstances and motivation to consider all aspects of personal experience and self-awareness. The following list is taken from a training course as to the 'group's' response to the question 'What is good mental health?'.

- Safety and well-being
- Respect
- Support networks and ability to maintain them
- Structured society
- Expressing emotions
- Ability to rationalize
- Manageable stress
- Culture
- Time for oneself
- Feeling valued
- Self-esteem
- Good relationships
- Having a role
- Confidence
- Enjoyment
- Control
- Contentment
- Assertiveness
- Happy childhood
- Physical health
- Friendship
- Socializing
- Financial security
- Peace of mind
- Stability in job,
- Home, relationships
- Feeling of belonging
- Ability to adapt to changes and stressors
- Choice/rights
- Degree of routine
- Variety
- Having realistic goals
- Sharing
- Support partners
- Good diet
- Love/belonging/ security
- Unloading problems
- Meaningful relationships/to be needed/loved
- Being considered rational in dealing with life events
- Being able to communicate in an honest way with others

- Having a satisfying sex life
- Being free of dependence on medication or illegal substances
- Achieving personal goals
- Ability to cope – use of coping mechanism
- Not being oppressed
- Personal–emotional development
- Self-love – self-worth – self-esteem – self-respect

This is obviously not definitive, and the discussion points can be used to enhance individual or group work.

Various discussion points can arise from considering this list:

1. What is missing from this list in relation to your own personal experience?
2. Can you develop this list in terms of your own language system for describing what constitutes good mental health?
3. Is there any way of prioritizing this list?
4. What are the foundational elements of mental health from the viewpoint of the 'public', 'professionals', and 'the state'?
5. What is the relationship between mental health and morality, if as children we require the right 'building blocks' to become neither mad nor bad?
6. How do you define the relationship between mental health and mental illness?

Health promotion

Given that developments in health promotion theory and practice have been informed by the Ottowa Charter (WHO 1986) we will begin our discussion with a common definition from the World Health Organization: 'Health promotion is the process of enabling people to increase control over, and to improve their health.' Goodstadt *et al.* (1987) extend this by describing health promotion as *the maintenance and enhancement of existing levels of health through the implementation of effective policies, programs and services.* (p.61). This places health promotion as directed towards the non-ill population. It also includes policies and programmes that increase or maintain health by using risk-avoidance or risk-reduction strategies. Achieving this requires the adoption of a social model of health recognizing an holistic and positive approach and highlighting sociocultural, economic, political and key environmental determinants of health. This provides an alternative to a traditional medical model addressing the symptoms rather than the causes of ill-health. It places medicine – or in our case psychiatry – in a

Compile a list of definitions of mental health from whatever sources you can.

Use them as discussion points with colleagues and clients.

wider societal context. This context acknowledges, accepts, and reveals the causes of ill-health and health inequalities as not the sole responsibility of individuals or health care services. They are the responsibility of a range of public and private organizations including national and local government. Health promotion incorporates three main elements within the broad context of a social model of health. This is described in more detail in Chapter 6 and briefly consists of:

- **Health education** – informing, influencing and empowering individuals and groups, communities and policy makers about the determinants of health and ways in which health may be preserved and improved
- **Prevention** – programmes and activities aimed at preventing ill-health, disease, accidents
- **Health protection** – encompassing a range of environmental, legal, fiscal, political, economic and social measures which promote health

This moves us away from a reductionist approach to health and broadens the debate to include identification of problems and possible solutions for promoting mental health.

A model for health

We now consider a model of health and more clearly identify some of the most important prerequisites. Foundations for mental health lie in the common humanity and expression of fundamental rights. This is true for all health as much as it is for our mental health. Adams and Pintus (1994) argue that to promote health requires a radical restructuring of society. They describe building blocks for health which include the following:

- Basic amenities – warmth, water supply, etc.
- Care
- Child care
- Education
- Freedom from violence and discrimination
- Housing
- Income
- Love
- Nutrition
- Safe working environment
- Sense of purpose and self-esteem
- Social rights

- Support (emotional/psychological/social)
- Sustainable development

Within this model health promotion is seen as having three aims:

1. To focus on these building blocks for health
2. To empower people and communities to extract the most out of systems
3. To empower collectively to challenge the structures that determine health experience.

These three aims can be achieved at various levels of intervention: policy, strategy, organizational, community and individual. How then might activity in the MHP field look? One approach is to look at some aims for promoting mental health and methods and action which could be developed as set out in Table 1.1.

Table 1.1 **Comprehensive approach to MHP?**	Aims	Method/action
	Improve community infrastructure	Engage with and support community development and community participation
	Support and develop coping strategies	Maximize opportunities for self-help on a range of mental health issues
	Make services more accessible	Enable contact and make services user-friendly and influenced by local needs
	Focus on prevention	Training and research-based preventive programmes
	Clarify professional roles and responsibilities	Audit of activity/SWOT analysis/ sharing other agencies' scope, limitation and philosophy of practice
	Sustain a matrix of contacts with agencies	Invest time and resources to identify and maintain a broad network of key stakeholders in the mental health and related fields
	Organize mental health resources more effectively	Plan according to service and 'felt needs'
	Educate the public	Provide information and contacts on mental health as well as mental ill-health

These aims need to be achieved with reference to an outer framework of anti-oppressive philosophy and practice. Meeting these aims also requires organizational development and training. A focus on the particular needs of specific groups, such as those experiencing poverty and discrimination, is one way forward. Such an approach can be refined further by tackling the issues within particular population groups (women, children, older adults) or in specific settings (primary care, hospitals, schools).

The need to tackle health – and mental health – inequalities, coupled with the importance of strategic alliances, continues to be viewed within the social domain by theorists in both health and social care. Bury *et al.* (1994) have recently examined the social causation of mental ill-health and possible interventions at various levels to combat mental illness and develop MHP. Their examination at four levels (individual, group, community and legislative) echoes the work of Whitehead (1995). They examined mental health promotion from a social model with a focus on several population groups: women, black and minority ethnic groups, and older adults.

The particular needs of other marginalized groups, those who are HIV positive for example, challenge the core of a social definition of health and mental health. Until the foundations of health – including the guiding principles from the Ottowa Charter enshrined in Health for All – are implemented, we can be said to have failed in addressing the mental and emotional health of individual groups and communities. Therefore, we will argue that fundamental issues are still not being addressed. The state makes rules on social and sexual conduct, on economic and environmental policy. These are political decisions that are of direct relevance to anyone's capacity for mental health. Part of the role of MHP must be to influence such decisions. This inevitably leads to a discussion of inequality in the field of mental health.

Inequality and mental health

Read and Wallcraft (1995) are clear in the relevance of inequality for our mental health:

> Inequality is bad for people's mental health. The discrimination and inequality that pervade life in 1990s Britain can fundamentally damage people's physical well-being, their confidence and their emotional health.

Recent guidelines jointly produced by MIND and Unison examine oppression and its relationship with mental distress and provide a range of recommendations with a focus on mental health service delivery. The problem of oppression is explored under the headings listed in Box 1.2. All of these are seen as having a negative effect on people's mental health. They impinge on the individual, their culture and community to prevent them from reaching and sustaining mental health. More importantly, oppression is seen as a cause of mental distress in itself. Who then experiences oppression? Oppression is difficult to define but is considered predominantly across a range of 'minority' groups including:

Oppressed citizens

- People with physical and sensory impairment
- Non-English speakers
- Older adults and young people
- Minority ethnic groups
- Lesbians, gay men
- Users and previous users of mental health services
- People with learning difficulties

Box 1.2 **Oppression**

- Discrimination
- Inequality
- Alienation
- Harassment
- Segregation
- Stereotyping

Psychiatric service provision, mental health policy and public perceptions and misconceptions can both perpetuate and reinforce oppression. As such, there is an opportunity for services to both identify and challenge such oppression which may contribute and continue to exacerbate a person's mental health problem. This is equally true of nonspecialist services, but increasingly the pressures on individuals to change organizational policy and practices in this way are too often outweighed by other pressing concerns, such as basic survival!

What solutions are proposed?

Read and Wallcraft (1995) call for genuine equal opportunity policies and programmes within the mental health arena and they include a detailed plan for the production and implementation of an equal opportunity policy. Many of the suggestions and solutions are practical and include training, choice for service users, awareness and sensitive responses to access, support groups within services, advocacy, information and involvement. Essentially, many of the contributions services can make are professional ones around openness, training and sensitivity. They are do-able tasks.

Health promotion – mental health – MHP: definitions

Although definitions can inhibit as well as encapsulate ideas, we need to reflect the range that surrounds health promotion and mental health. Such definitions exist within a dynamic range of influences and as such are open to change and evolution. Environmental issues, for example, have recently come to the political foreground, with international policy and local decision making on Agenda 21 (United Nations Conference on Environment and Development (UNCED) 1992) highlighting the need for action on sustainable development. Within our local practice in Sheffield, a broad definition of health promotion has developed taking account of such shifts in thinking and practice:

A broad definition of health promotion

The promotion of health is concerned with the maximizing of individual's and communities' involvement in improving and protecting the quality of life and well-being. Health promotion aims to address equity in health, the risks to health, sustainable environment conducive to health, and the empowerment of individuals and communities by contributing to healthy public policy, advocating for health, enabling skills development and education.

(Sheffield Health Promotion 1996)

This broad definition of health promotion is essential if we are to consider mental health as broader than psychiatry and mental health services. Aside from being one of the first health promotion units to predate Health of the Nation by appointing a Health Promotion Specialist for MHP, Sheffield has been a focus for MHP activity. This has included a Healthy City approach to mental and emotional well-being, championing of community-focused initiatives, provider development, purchasing of MHP, evaluation, training and curriculum influences. An early attempt to define MHP was produced by a multi-agency group comprising voluntary and statutory agencies in health and social care planning and provision. The following definition was used by this group to clarify aims and rationale.

What is mental health promotion?

Mental health promotion is developing positive mental health both for and with the community in general and individuals who may have mental health problems. It includes self-help, service provision and organizational skills.

> The concept of mental health promotion recognizes that an individual's mental health is inextricably linked with their relationship to others, their lifestyle, and the environmental factors that affect that, and the degree of power they can exert over their lives.
>
> (Sheffield Mental Health Promotion Group 1992)

Despite the introduction of mental illness as a key area of The Health of the Nation (DOH 1993a), and an acknowledgement that MHP is a vehicle for meeting targets, difficulties remain. MHP has not had the infrastructure, profile or development work other areas have had, such as accident prevention and coronary heart disease health promotion programmes. The Mental Health Task Force was established to initiate innovative practice, although this has tended to focus on improving mental health service provision. More recently, the Health Education Authority (HEA) has taken over responsibility for coordinating activity as part of World Mental Health Day. It is also in the process of developing core indicators to help evaluate mental health promotion. In its recent literature several definitions of mental health and MHP are given. Each has a slightly different focus. These are described in Table 1.2.

Table 1.2 **Mental health: definition and focus**	Definition	Focus
	One way of describing mental health is that it is the emotional resilience which enables us to enjoy life and survive pain, disappointment and sadness. It is a positive sense of well-being and an underlying belief in our own, and others' dignity and worth. (Mental Health Factsheet, Health Education Authority 1996)	The focus here is mental health as a protective force underpinned by a collective responsibility to others.
	Mental health is described as including a range of capacities which emphasizes our potential for growth, change and social nature. (*Together we Stand*, DOH 1995a)	The emphasis is developmental and of maintaining and sustaining skills.
(continued opposite)	*Much is already being attempted in local communities. We consider that a health promotion strategy would want to identify the best of these and to devise means that help provide them with support, encouragement and appropriate evaluation, as well as enabling similar projects to be attempted elsewhere. Whether this*	MHP as a vehicle for change at the individual, community and structural levels – a bottom-up approach. This is clearly referring to a community development approach to promoting mental health.

(continued opposite)

Definition	Focus	Table 1.2 **Mental health: definition and focus** (*continued*)
strategy focuses on broad based public campaigns, professional training, or on health education, its best chances of success must surely come by maximising involvement 'from the bottom up'. (Bury *et al.* 1994, p.31)		
To enable people to manage life events, both predictable and unpredictable, through the enhancement of self-esteem and a sense of well-being. To achieve this through working with individuals, groups and communities to improve life-skills and the quality of life. (Mental Health Priorities for Action, Executive Summary HEA internal document, Greenoak *et al.* 1994)	The intention is to manage and control circumstances through bolstering self-esteem.	

These statements and definitions reflect the importance of community-focused as well as individual-focused activity in promoting mental health. This approach is now considered more explicitly.

Community

Much could be said about the relevance of 'community' in any analysis and debate of mental health promotion, but we can only touch on the most salient points from our perspective. As our identification is one that we hope might lead to more positive action within this arena, it has to be up to each individual to appreciate the commitment inherent in doing this, and to acquire more knowledge and experience where they can, especially in terms of how this might lead to 'good practice'. Tudor (1996) in his recent book on MHP, explores the notion of community mental health promotion as a ' . . . concept and practice in its own right' (p.109). He provides a useful critique of the sources from which a vision of community MHP could be realized.

The importance of 'sociological' mental health practice, and in this a realization of the positives and negatives of 'therapy'.

The increase in value that has to be given to user-led involvement and initiatives within a defined framework which assists, not prevents, people in the 'community' to challenge the stigmatizing nature of mental illness and to promote their mental health.

Debates about 'community', in its myriad forms, will continue to be a focus of struggle and opposing ideologies. Our main interest and concern, within a 'health for all' framework, has to be how people relate to one another in all aspects of social participation, specifically within a locality where identified structures are in place to support our psychological, spiritual, sociocultural and economic needs and wants, whether we choose to call that 'community' or not. This is the minefield: the residence, the street, the local neighbourhood, the village, the town, the city, the county, where so much diversity is contained, and the source of such unequal distribution of welfare and opportunity is manifested. The euphemism these days for having an unmarried partner is 'living together'. Maybe the word 'community' should be replaced by this term. If you truly 'live with' someone, you have decided to accept differences, you are able to give and take, to love in the sense of being free to do so, and to look to the future not the past in any healthy developmental process. In terms of our mental health, we perhaps need to hold constantly in our minds two levels of interpretation: the fact that we have 'everyday' mental health needs within the social world we inhabit at any given time; and the relational–foundational elements that determine our ability to engage in these in the first place. We are aware of the circularity or 'dialectic' inherent in this process. We expect, because other people do so, to be able to participate in work, family life, leisure and social pursuits and to do this from a platform of having our basic health and safety needs met. This is obviously not the case. If thousands of us are being killed off prematurely through stress and illness because we do work, and the highest incidence of abuse, homicide and violence occur in familial settings, it would seem overdue that we consider these issues more explicitly.

'Community' is the concept that gives vision to a network of relationships which strike at the very heart of our wants and desires. However much information technology, the Internet, the world of second-hand or virtual experience, assuage some of our baser requirements, there is a point where we cannot escape engaging with others, and it is a sad indictment of any society that our communities are so full of paedophiles, rapists, and abusers of women and children and elderly people and property. We also know that there are abusive parents, teachers, therapists, doctors, nurses and social workers, and the list could go on. We cannot ignore an unconscious element in our understanding of mental health problems, or mental illness, or the power differentials that exists in relation to community living. We will always have to consider how our mental health needs are constituted over and above our 'basic instincts' as children or adults.

The carving up of a community's health and social welfare needs into an artificially manufactured profit zone is one of the saddest and most disheartening manifestations of over 17 years of dominant conservative values. Enshrined in us all is our potential to satisfy the demand for private and individual profit at the most vulnerable times of our life. Whether we reside in statutory or private facilities, such as children's homes, mental health units, secure units, special hospitals, prisons, or elderly care provision, we know that 'balancing the books' takes more and more precedence over common sense and cooperative and comprehensive services. Our examination of mental health problems in the community has also to be considered in the light of the very real dilemma thousands of people are facing in terms of illness as disability, and the economic and social problems being experienced by them and those who care for them.

> For one thing, the whole language in which the new dispensation is cast is Tory-speak, market-speak. Providers, users, purchasers, consumers. It is the language of the market-place, denoting the language of money. The one place in an individualistic, selfish, self-seeking society where people matter, where use value and not exchange value is paramount, is now being turned into an accountant's playground. (Sivanandan 1993, p.34)

If we extend the debate about community more specifically in relation to people who are mentally ill, there would seem to be three identified areas of concern: how policies are being implemented; the 'substance' of these policies; and the principles upon which they are based (Dalley 1996, p.8). Since we began writing this book the government has renamed care in the community as 'comprehensive mental health services'. This rephrasing is timely, as more and more people are finding out how little statutory responsibility there is for community care: there are increasing numbers of people being imprisoned, and fewer statutory beds for the mentally ill. The statistics for 1996 are that 1000 more places are required each month in line with new sentencing policies. There is also an increase in the incidence of those with serious mental health problems being held in prison and an increase in the need for 'treatment' orders in special hospitals, regional secure units and acute in-patient facilities. From 1980 until 1994 the number of hospital beds fell by half, and there is currently a crisis in inner-city areas, especially London which is having to be tackled in terms of crisis intervention and concentration of resources on those registered as dangerous and 'at risk' (Audit Commission 1994).

The whole climate in which any real assessment of our mental health needs, in terms of community mental health, can be made has been all too easily sidetracked, for the economic reasons identified and in the ideological world which is built on fear, narrow 'scientific' thinking, person-blaming, family-blaming and above all a desire for retribution. The high profile for locking people up because they are a danger to themselves and any local community where they might be placed might be a necessity now but, as with many of the present policies, it has short-term benefit. The principles inherent in dominant conservative ideology are apparent in the way the onus of responsibility has shifted so dramatically towards individual and groups in the informal, private and voluntary sectors of any given community. The position of carers is also well documented in Dalley's book on community and collectivism. She extends her analysis to consider very closely the position of female and male carers in our society. Our understanding, within an exploration of a framework for community mental health promotion, could not be comprehensive without an examination of feminist approaches to more democratic policy-making, relevant theory, research, ethical practice and dialogue (Hugman and Smith 1995; Payne 1991). It is perhaps to social work that mental health nurses should be looking if they wish to enhance their knowledge in this domain and in terms of anti-oppressive practice; there are currently many texts which would support theoretical and practice needs and identified outcomes.

From a broader perspective, have we completely abandoned collective or socialist values because they are too idealistic or unattainable and always have been? Or is it more important to tinker with language to make things more palliative in the political or professional arena and to continue to ignore the obvious? Is it at all possible to hold universalistic values, considering the cultural context of community participation in modern-day society? Has economic 'necessity' got such a grip on us that we have lost sight of positive attributes and attitudes, such as authenticity, respect, integrity and compassion? How much importance are we as nurses placing on ethical practice that is about use value and not exchange value in our involvement with people in the community, where mental health nursing has a high profile and involvement? In social work this fundamental dilemma has had much more exposure (Humphries 1996). Again we have an example of how much more collaboration needs to take place in terms of community involvement in health and social care. We need to break down many barriers to do this, not only among relevant 'professionals' but with the people whose care and emotional well-being depend on them. Community mental health promotion has to maintain this focus.

MHP as a community-focused activity

Money (1996) also identifies 'the community' as central to developing positive mental health. He sees it as essential to clarify the difference between mental health and mental illness, treatment, prevention and promotion. This should be done through a broad approach and a range of activity. Five dimensions for MHP are described – individual, interpersonal, power locus, environmental and therapeutic:

- **Individual.** Positive community mental health as a measure of its success: focus on positive states, freedom from crime, community-originated solutions
- **Interpersonal.** Community structures supporting interpersonal relationships. A family focus: voluntary groups, local politics, religion, and a maximum participation in decision making
- **Power locus.** Maximize internal locus of control – sense of control, grassroots democracy, devolving decision making processes, local neighbourhood control
- **Environmental.** A healthy environment: reduced pollution, open spaces, traffic free areas, safe play areas for children, lighting, safety
- **Therapeutic.** Health care which is accessible, flexible and offers choice and is focused upon prevention as well as nonmedical interventions; also includes sport, leisure, etc.

The work of Money, when placed against the model of health by Adams and Pintus (1994), can offer a blueprint for a community-focused approach to MHP. What they both embrace is the importance of local needs, wants and aspirations as well as accommodating the importance for the expertise of specialists and generic services. They also serve to stress the impact that government policy and agency at the national and international levels have on achieving and sustaining mental health. In short, what is required for the promotion of positive mental and emotional well-being is a combination of action at the level of citizens, services and the state.

Towards a framework. Development of our definition for MHP

From the range of definitions of mental health and its promotion given, we now consider the level of analysis necessary for our identification of MHP.

The public

The public as individuals, groups and communities has traditionally seen mental health as a negative phenomenon more associated with illness than health. The stigma surrounding mental illness is shrouded in myth and controversy and, as with other matters of illness, people have historically been the passive recipients of treatment. Although there is a long way to go, services have become more responsive to the needs of an increasingly assertive and informed public. People are also recognizing that other factors need to be in place to maintain mental health. The public's perception of mental health includes their environment, social support and employment. Mental ill-health is also seen as wider than a dominant model of psychiatry suggests and includes stress, relationship problems, poverty and discrimination. This provides us with an initial definition of what MHP attempts to realize:

> *To promote mental health in this area is to see a general improvement in the standards of community infrastructure as well as support and coping strategies at the interpersonal level.*

Mental health can be promoted and sustained by action at the social level, improving the fabric of and access to housing, transport, training, employment, leisure and opportunities for informal support. Skills and opportunities for community and self-reliance can be improved at the individual and community levels. This can range from self-help, community and voluntary groups to specific locally inspired activity on health-related issues, such as a lobby group for responding to a drugs problem on an estate.

Health and social care professionals

The dominant role played by mental health professionals has led to a range of specialties. Their approach and methodologies results in service delivery provided, primarily, at the individual level. Practice has focused on dysfunction and treatment to ameliorate the distress of certain standardized conditions. A move from institutional care and treatment, and concepts such as normalization, have resulted in a change in emphasis towards community mental health. This move has at times led to a degree of exploitation rather than partnership with the non-service sector. The geographic location of services and specialties may have changed, but not so much in the way of their philosophy and practice. However, the social realities which impact on the communities that professionals serve should begin to influence their role and responses. General practice fundholding and the contract culture are also factors which professionals will need to respond to with other agencies if they are to cope with mental health as well as mental illness. MHP for the community psychiatric nurse (CPN), the social worker or the health visitor is about boundaries and territory. Practitioners need to know what they do and what they cannot do in order to enable them to discover why they do it. It is in this process that they can build up the layers and complexity of practice which release them from the captivity of professionalism. This leads to our second definition of MHP:

> *To promote mental health in this area is to make services more accessible, focus on prevention and recognize professional limitations and the skills and potential of other statutory and nonstatutory agencies.*

The process by which services are made more accessible is a critical step in a mental health-promoting way of working. It requires not only refinement of what, where and when services are delivered, but also of who and how this can be determined. The involvement of users and carers and of other stakeholders in the mental health field is of vital importance here. Professionals also have power to influence and advocate and are in a good position to deliver preventive policy and strategy for mental health as much as for mental illness.

The state

Cost is a major factor for any government in relation to health and social care provision. This is as true of nations with more privately oriented approaches to health as it is to the United Kingdom. Health gain and outcome measurement, resource prioritization, cost-effectiveness and quality have all been high on political agendas in the Western world. Unemployment, crime and family breakdown (cause and effect of mental ill-health) are also political agenda setters. So are the expectations of voters, who attach significance to the need for interventionist policies and programmes to tackle these issues. The state and its systems recognize the key role health and social care have to play in this area. Therefore, a range of targets, health strategies and programmes have been developed to counter the increasing demands put on budgets. As with the professionals' focus on health, the state tends to see health as an individual responsibility. This can result in promoting mental health as improving existing health services and the idea that people 'look after' their emotional health. Public health education, as opposed to health promotion, is the preferred approach. Such a focus gives us our third definition of MHP:

> *To promote mental health in this area is to organize current mental health resources more effectively and to educate the public to be aware of their role in being mentally well.*

These three broad areas and definitions give an indication of the different outcomes for promoting mental health which the public, professionals and the state see as important. It is also necessary to recognize these desired outcomes when looking critically at what is meant by mental health promotion. This text considers these three themes at the political as well as the practical levels.

This enables us to produce a definition of our own which is a synthesis of the perceptions and tensions that exist about mental health, mental illness and its promotion and prevention between the public, professional agencies and the state:

Mental health promotion is the action element of any comprehensive interpretation of everyone's mental health needs and wants. It is underpinned by an anti-oppressive framework for practice which emphasizes cooperative social participation. This is fundamental in realistically addressing the conflictual nature of relationships between the public, professionals and the state. (Boxer and McCulloch 1996)

A structure for action

Our review and examination of the literature and models so far reveals common themes. These are listed in Box 1.3. Individuals, communities, agencies and policy makers all have a contribution to make in these areas. With the right combination the task is not only achievable but the process itself can become health enhancing. There are risks that need to be taken and views and opinions can become entrenched. However, the process by which this can be achieved need not prove the ideological struggle of competing viewpoints. There is a common ground: we all require mentally healthy communities; without them we descend into chaos.

Box 1.3 **Comon themes identified in MHP**

1. The need to reduce stress at the individual, community and organizational level
2. The need to educate and raise awareness on positive mental health as well as mental illness
3. The need for community development, for locally inspired solutions
4. The need for a user and carer focus to support their mental and emotional health needs
5. The need for prevention, especially in the areas of depression, suicide and self-harm

Practice points

Thinking Ahead (Braidwood 1995) consisted of a national review of MHP strategies and came up with eight criteria for practice:

- Empowerment
- A strategic approach
- A public health basis
- Theory basis
- Health promotion basis
- Positive health

How far can your practice meet these criteria?

- Researched basis
- Alliances

Elements of a framework for mental health promotion

Context

We now consider more closely a framework that can inform practice in the field of mental health promotion. Tudor, in his recent text, emphasizes elements of what is needed for positive mental health and attempts to fit them to a theoretical framework for mental health promotion (see Box 1.4).

Box 1.4 **Practice elements**

- Coping
- Tension and stress management
- Self-concept and identity
- Self-esteem
- Self-development
- Autonomy
- Change
- Social support and movement

(Tudor 1996, p.63)

However important these factors are, the emphasis would seem to be that they appear to reside more in a socio-psychological, rather than socio-economic–political domain. This translation, in Tudor's account, does not provide the requirements for practice that we use as a core element. In identifying the relationship between public, professionals and the state, we place greater importance and value in anti-oppressive practice as being a requirement which intertwines with MHP at all levels. In the current political climate, anti-oppressive practice does not have value and is seen as 'ideologically laden', negated by incorrect interpretation of political correctness and having no real place in social care education and training (Dominelli, 1997a; Hugman and Smith, 1995; Humphries, 1996). Our identification of MHP is that its purpose is to promote a realistic approach to welfare issues, and to do this 'existing power differentials' between and within diverse groups of people have to be challenged. Dalrymple and Burke (1995) map out quite clearly their framework for anti-oppressive practice (Box 1.5).

Box 1.5 Suggested framework for anti-oppressive practice

- Personal self-knowledge
- Knowledge and an understanding of the majority social systems
- Knowledge and understanding of different groups and cultures
- Knowledge of how to challenge and confront issues on a personal and structural level
- Awareness of the need to be 'research minded' (Everitt *et al.* 1992)
- Commitment to action and change

(Dalrymple and Burke 1995, p.18)

We consider that the knowledge and skills required in mental health nursing form much of the basis of our realization of a framework for mental health promotion, but without a foundational element as there is in social work theory and practice (Dalrymple and Burke 1995). If there is any time when mental health nurses should act as positive role models, then for the future of this branch of nursing and the development of community services it is now. No one can undertake such a role without acknowledgment of the historical development and continuation of oppressive psychiatric practices. As many of the 'hands on' skills required in traditional training are being undertaken by carers or health and social care assistants, there is an urgent need for an educative role or facilitation by trained staff who can provide the 'rationale' for doing so and the development of cooperative practice. How can we achieve this? Obviously we will not be able to do very much while we remain steeped in selective memory loss and 'obfuscation', for example with regard to the early days of race-awareness training and why it was so important (Patel 1995). Although we have considered the spectrum of oppression and our work has been to encourage self-reflection about all oppressed 'groups', the link to disadvantage because of the colour of one's skin is still paramount. In a recent article in the *Nursing Times*, concerns about racism within nursing and the health service are seen as adversely affecting people's mental health, especially because discrimination is so rife and has a knock-on effect in terms of 'staff morale, reputation and making the best use of available resources' (Mensah 1996). This author cites a very recent experience in the classroom of a school of nursing while teaching about antidiscriminatory practice, when one of the black nurse's in the class recounted that she had:

. . . recently experienced the wrath of her ward manager who had admonished: 'You're an immigrant – get that chip off your shoulder. Stop complaining or go home to Africa.' – That to a third-generation British black woman who had only ever travelled as far as Scotland. (Mensah 1996, p.26)

Just as there is a problem in how one uses differing theoretical accounts to inform knowledge and competent practice, we must ask whether we really have a commitment to changing our attitudes and practices so that the core problematics of social interaction are not also oppressive and damaging and to realize this as being fundamental to positive mental health and personal and professional relationships (Patel 1995). The many relationships we make, such as doctor–nurse, doctor/nurse–patient, social worker–client, are difficult enough without the added dimension of 'racism' in its most blatant form affecting the emotional well-being of those experiencing it. As an emerging vision of practice in health and social care there is a general consensus from those working within this domain that anti-oppressive practice and critical education are the way forward (Dominelli 1997a; Humphries 1996). Anti-oppressive practice considers the whole spectrum of 'oppressed' experience, and does not work on the principle of berating people for the mistakes of their ancestors. What we have to deal with are the very obvious wrongs that are still happening now and which can inform better working relationships if handled sensitively and pragmatically. Social work, through key initiatives from people working at the interface of theory and practice, embraces this concept, however complex, but nursing is still coming to grips with key changes in emphasis and understanding (Ahmad 1990).

Feminist practice

If there is one place where the personal and the political collide, it is within oppressive mental health practice. We consider that there are important links to the development of anti-oppressive practice in feminist theory and practice. This forms part of our framework for education and training in mental health promotion, however limited our consideration has had to be within the remit of this book.

> Gender is invisible in much mainstream research and policy making. This does not mean that policies and practice are neutral as far as gender is concerned. In a world where sexist ideologies which reinforce male power dominate, gender blindness means that women's needs are often simply not recognized, or worse, derided. (Barnes and Maple 1992, p.141)

As is highlighted in other chapters, the identification of one gendered half of the population as having such a higher incidence of mental health problems, and being deemed 'vulnerable', is a major problematic. To some extent this has been alleviated by anything other than mainstream practice and has been a source of much discouragement and negative approaches to women and their mental health needs (Dalley 1996). Arguments about biology and destiny have a strong hold in both biomedical and psychodynamic approaches and, whatever their validity, no unaware person would deny the 'oppressions' that dominate all but a few women and which are still not being addressed at the level of practice. Consideration of black women's mental health has so far been a neglected aspect of the debate, as the 'problem' with young black men has given psychiatry one of its biggest challenges to further categorize 'mental illness'. Feminist counselling has been the bedrock of informed approaches to practice but is not an integral part of the teaching of interpersonal skills in health and social care courses (Dominelli and McLeod 1992).

Anti-oppressive practice

Definition of anti-oppressive practice

Anti-oppressive practice aims to provide more appropriate and sensitive services by responding to people's needs regardless of their social status. AOP embodies a person-centred philosophy; an egalitarian value system concerned with reducing the deleterious effects of structural inequalities upon people's lives; a methodology focusing on both process and outcome; and a way of structuring relationships between individuals that aims to empower users by reducing the negative effects of hierarchy on their interactions and the work they do together.

(Dominelli 1997a, p.24)

Anti-oppressive practice and the development of therapeutic relationships are intertwined, however much that practice, especially within statutory provision, is full of conflict and contradiction. Unless the foundations of work and experience in this area are considered at the level of both policy and practice, and we have highlighted reasons why this might be not be the case, nothing will really change. If we consider the high proportion of people who have mental health problems, not just in terms of vulnerability through the life-cycle, but in terms of the disabling 'ism's' which are superimposed, there are still many unanswered questions.

We have encountered many people who ask for concreteness in our emphasis on mental health promotion as a viable construct which can be 'taught'. We consider that they are missing the point. There is no 'magic' from this perspective, just a lot of hard work, soul searching, and an acceptance that what people hold on to in terms of their prejudices and intolerance has to do with beliefs and attitudes which can change given the right circumstances and motivation. Anyone working in this field should have this motivation; it is more than a job. It has to be considered in terms of the accountability and responsibility we have to our fellow human beings as a result of earning a salary off the backs of their problems and disadvantages.

> *Promoting emotional and social well-being is not possible without a framework which at the moment is best represented by anti-oppressive practice.*

There are a small number of key texts which address anti-oppressive practice and which consider that it is also necessary to gain insight into what constitutes antiracist and antidiscriminatory policy and practice. It is perhaps not enough just to know what dates are important in terms of equal opportunities policies, however much the law and the administration of it affect our daily lives. Professor Dominelli has written extensively on the subject of antiracist, anti-oppressive practice, especially within social work education, and Thompson's (1993) book on antidiscriminatory practice gives a useful overview. Other writers such as Dalrymple and Burke (1995) provide an account of anti-oppressive practice from the perspective of social care and the law which is also very informative and accessible to students and practitioners wanting to develop reflexive knowledge when working with children or people who have mental health problems or learning disabilities. Obviously there are more texts relevant to this subject than we have been able to consider. We hope that if people, especially students, are committed to changing bad practice in health and social care settings, they will consider this approach as the basis of 'good practice' and become better informed and involved in this process.

It is paramount that there can be a translation into practice and we hope that if people are really interested in the promotion of mental health they will find out from their academic institution or practice area what is happening in this field and encourage as much positive dialogue and debate as they can. Any teaching we have undertaken in mental health promotion to date has been underpinned by our commitment to anti-oppressive practice, and in our relationships with people we have grown wiser and stronger from this. At the time of writing we are aware of one positive initiative linking a local black mental health agency with one of the special hospitals.

Empowerment and anti-oppressive practice

The concept of empowerment is an important element in our understanding of how we can counter oppression, and in reflecting the

Is it the case that services have to develop in an apartheid system where only black people can effectively provide the care for black people, and white people for white people, Asian people by other Asian people? Is there a context in which, across cultures, we can provide care for each other? What factors prevent this? How do agencies identify and offer support to people who are categorized as 'mixed race' or 'other'?

paradoxical position of mental health practice and what is wrong with so much of it. Humphries (1996), in her recent book on the subject, considers empowerment to have very strong positive and negative dimensions in both education and practice concerns. Dalrymple and Burke (1995), in developing a model for anti-oppressive practice, consider the process of empowerment to include the need for 'biography', rather than assessment, in terms of levels of feelings, ideas, activity, changed consciousness and political action (p.54). These authors provide a comprehensive account of the inherent dilemmas at the level of micro- and macro-analysis of theory and practice. The more traditionalist in nursing might consider this approach too abstract or partial in its application to practice goals. An example might be that, with the recent changes to the Mental Health Act in terms of concurrent hospital and prison orders, the motivation by 'professionals' to empower patients becomes confused. This is highlighted at a micro-level with the importance placed on 'individual' responsibility. At a macro-level, do we make it a goal to help people empower themselves because we and they are in the right circumstances to do so, or do we assume that the power and domination of welfare ideology are overwhelming (Humphries 1996).

One of the main themes in our reading about oppression is that we need to start with ourselves in the context of our personal and professional experience, which is still very ill-defined in much of psychiatric practice.

Student-centred approach

For students who have an opportunity to engage in learning about anti-oppressive, empowering or liberating practice there are major concerns which need to be made explicit. This means that education providers really have to change the emphasis away from accepting ill-defined notions of student-centred or experiential learning, reducing educational experience to how many students can be fitted into an ill-equipped environment, or using ill-designed curricula and traditional Eurocentric educational approaches. Obviously, within the current economic climate that is very difficult and frustrating for both teachers and students, who often know what is needed to improve things.

If anything can be achieved as a student it is to be treated primarily as an equal partner in the quest for experiential knowledge, hopefully within the framework of a tripartite system of supervision in academic institutions and practice settings. Obviously, personal limitations and problems exist, and it would be naive to ignore the very nature of being a student and the varying reactions to this. In identifying and encouraging self-management and a sound value base to practice, students have a key role to play in the development of both anti-oppressive practice and MHP (Dominelli 1997a).

The main areas to consider might range over the following:

- Developing innovative practice objectives
- Contributing to group development, indicative content and debate
- Writing essays and assignments which cover more controversial practice issues
- Being a change-agent in determining better or more equitable service provision
- Level of awareness about self and others

One of the key problems for students is providing educators and practitioners with the necessary evaluation of their performance and their 'right' to be considered an expert or professional. This change is long overdue in nursing, where hierarchical relationships and emphasis of management status continue to oppress many people. Some of these key points are summed up by Professor Dominelli in determining any course philosophy and learning outcomes for course content in health and social care education (Box 1.6).

Box 1.6 **What is anti-oppressive practice?**

A course's commitment to Anti-Oppressive Practice is not mere ideological baggage. It is rooted in both life experience and research . . . To begin with, students learn better in small groups than in large ones. Having small groups in which to teach AOP is essential if we are to pay due attention to process and outcome. Many of the issues that are addressed in AOP call forth strong emotions and much controversy as we struggle to integrate theory with practice and personal growth. Students need to understand themselves as well as the issues placed before them. Doing this calls for reflective introspection as well as action. Effective AOP requires the integration of intellectual, emotional and practical knowledge which best occurs through very small group discussions which can proceed at the student's own pace rather than according to a pre-determined timetable. Students who attempt to work in anti-oppressive ways cannot rely on the imposition of dogma. They have to possess infinite capacities for mature and critical assessments which require the integration of technical professional knowledge and skills with a deep understanding of how individuals and society create and maintain a variety of social relationships and a commitment to promoting equality and respect for individual well-being. 'Political Correctness' therefore has no place in Anti-Oppressive Practice. Indeed, it is a travesty and a mockery of it. (Dominelli 1997a, p.28)

Participation

Nurses have found it difficult to develop a strategic role in health promotion, let alone MHP. Apart from basic requirements, such as a health visiting role with children and families, many of the therapeutic and health-promoting elements of past nursing practice are, both in hospitals and in the community, being handed over to the voluntary and private sectors while health and social care 'professionals' squabble over conceptual and practice territories. Within mental health services, the way mental health promotion has been realized has so far been piecemeal and has tended to duplicate a medical–lifestyle approach, even though 'nurses make up the largest professional group supporting people who have mental health problems' (Brooker *et al.* 1996, p.12). The overlap in terms of core skills or requirements for mental health nurses very much mirrors the requirements for mental health social work. There is still considerable work being undertaken which considers interdisciplinary education and training as being paramount, and in educational circles is trying to identify a new 'mental health worker' or what is understood by generic and specialist practice. An important and emerging aspect of current mental health practice is development of partnerships with users or ex-users of services, and we have highlighted this in terms of more recent educational approaches and 'good practice', as we do in other chapters. *OpenMind* (the bi-monthly journal from MIND) provides an invaluable source of publications and developments from this perspective.

Our identification of a framework would require everyone to participate and would highlight the problem of where and how we start to do this, especially with the critical relationship that exists between the public, professionals and the state. It would seem that instances of personal tragedy, and the way these are highlighted by the media are sometimes the only impetus for changes in policy and practice that occur so quickly and usually without agreement from those from different theoretical and political persuasions. The incident at Dunblane School and the death of head teacher Stephen Lawrence in 1996, and the deaths of a small number of people at the hands of psychiatric patients or disturbed individuals in the community, have focused attention on our morality and, although this is always understated, our mental health needs as being inextricably bound up in this. Calls for a 'moral referendum' would need to consider how much priority is given to mental health as inextricably linked to our capabilities as rational human beings to be able to adhere to a moral code of conduct in the first place. When do we start more openly encouraging people to consider their mental health needs from a moral and practical standpoint?

Professionals all too easily become aware how ethical codes for practice and conduct conflict with the obvious constraints that 'situated experience' engenders.

Framework for mental health promotion

We now identify a framework for education/training and practice, as envisaged so far, and consider more closely how this could be integrated into mainstream mental health practice. As discussed, the 'where', 'how' and 'why' of education have to be considered in a developing process which concentrates on human interaction as much as it does on content and the notion of having to 'teach' something. This is not to say that we can ignore the need for identified competence; for example, to be highly empathic in utilizing caring and enabling skills; to achieve the right blend of theory and practice; and to understand what can and cannot be achieved in this respect. Our definition of mental health promotion underpins the very 'nature' of our framework (Box 1.7).

Box 1.7 **Core elements for the theory and practice of MHP**

- Anti-oppressive practice
- Empowerment of self and others
- Self-awareness/reflection at the level of the personal and professional commitment given to the above
- Holistic interpretation
- Cooperative/social practice
- Therapeutic/feminist practice
- Ethical practice
- Sound knowledge of the subject
- Experiential and person-centred approaches to learning
- Continuous development and refinement of knowledge and practice

---

As this is a developing field, the emphasis on these aspects has to be at the level of participation in dialogue, in interpretation and in informing competence. For example, you might consider that you are already working within the above framework to the best of your ability and that other people are completely unaware of this! The identification of what constitutes 'competence' in relation to statutory practice, and why it is so important, should not detract from the above, but it usually does. We consider that the primary focus of our framework centres on the following:

1. The well-being of the people with whom we have contact
2. More balance between therapeutic and economic relationship
3. Being proactive rather than reactive
4. Empowering not oppressing
5. Experiential and person-centred approaches to learning.

Conclusions

This has been a difficult chapter to write. It is not easy to capture the essence of mental health promotion from our perspective. Our central concern is more than 'things are not the way they used to be'; they were never very good in the first place! The development of mainstream mental health services has never been a healthy one. There will always be those who think that it is every person for themselves, and that only in extreme crisis should anyone intervene in another person's affairs to this degree. The emergence of service users' voices testifying that after experiencing mainstream services they would probably agree with that attitude is a realistic indictment, yet we feel that much has been and could be achieved. There is an indefinable boundary between mental health and illness and our consideration has therefore to be broad-based, realistic and eclectic. We do not see mental health promotion as some kind of new 'religion', and we are aware that there might be some difficulty in realizing, or acting on, fundamental religious beliefs with the approach we have taken. This is especially true in relationships between women and men, and we write this at a time when many of the gains made by women, in describing the actual reality of their experiences, and identified in theory and practice concerns, are still not incorporated into mainstream approaches. We return to many of the issues raised in this chapter throughout the book and consider them more closely from a variety of perspectives. Our main aim is that what has been written is further 'food for thought' as to how we might raise the profile of our own and others' mental health if that realization will see an end to unnecessary and undesirable oppressive practices and unacceptable inequality between the 'us' and 'them' of this world.

Consider carefully your own account of what the author is saying in Box 1.6. You may find it interesting to argue the case for and against anti-oppressive practice, over other approaches to these issues, in health and social care education, with colleagues or with other students.

Discuss the points raised with your teachers and colleagues.

How could this approach be incorporated within your course framework?

The dimensions of oppression include race, gender, age, disability, class and sexual orientation: Where do you place yourself in this?

Analyse any relationship that could exist between them which could further compound oppressive experience.

Consider a global context to this in relation to economic, cultural and social experience.

How far are you prepared to discuss any of the above with people who define themselves as oppressed in the ways highlighted, including your family, colleagues, managers, 'professionals', users, ex-users of services?

Do you consider that mental health promotion and anti-oppressive practice are the 'democratic' and fundamental elements of health and social care education, training and practice?

Try to clarify your understanding of the framework for MHP suggested above:

- Discuss with as many people as possible how this might be incorporated into mainstream mental health education and training;
- Can these elements be translated into defined competence or are they just ideals within an unclear value-base to practice?
- How can this framework for practice be incorporated into the objectives and indicative content of health and social care courses?
- How can this framework inform better relationships between professionals, service-users and the wider public in promoting our mental health?
- What research and development are you aware of which could inform this framework?

2

Mental health promotion and the policy context

Mental health promotion . . . entails an inherently political strategy, which targets social and material aspects of society. It is also an approach which envisages the involvement of other groups of people apart from medical professionals. (Rogers and Pilgrim 1996, p.146)

Key themes:

- Significant mental 'health' policy
- Healthy public policy
- Health and social care policy and the professions
- State policy

Overview

All health and social policy is significant in the realm of MHP. As Tones and Tilford (1994) highlight, health promotion is a synergy between health education and healthy public policy. The prevention of mental illness and the promotion of mental health are only possible if environmental, fiscal, economic and social policies are in place to support the basic foundations for health. Whether they relate to jobs, training, accommodation or equal opportunities they are all vital parts for a mentally healthy society, or otherwise. They influence the foundations for health and ultimately its promotion.

A policy is a statement of what should happen at the strategic, intermediate and operational levels. A range of policy directly and indirectly has had an impact on mental illness services and the potential for mental health over the last century. Essentially, policy involves formal decisions and actions, is about implementation, and is refined over time.

Significant policy

Peckham (1996), in a recent review of policy developments, recognizes the considerable shifts that have occurred and are continuing to take place in the NHS. Their impact reveals itself in various reports and strategies which have incorporated these new policy developments. The Butterworth report (Butterworth 1994), for example, anticipates that the practitioner will act as resource allocator, coordinator, clinician, educator and illness preventer; all this while forming and maintaining a variety of networks and contacts. These are the ingredients for potential MHP practice, but they require other policies in place to be performed competently.

What are the key ingredients of contemporary health and social policy which have a bearing on MHP?

Given the nature of current policy and its dynamic status, a definitive response to this question cannot be confidently provided. However, there are themes in contemporary health and social care policy that recur (Box 2.1).

Box 2.1 **Policy themes in health and social care**

- Deinstitutionalization, with a move from hospital to community care
- A division between purchasers and providers of health and social care
- A focus for achieving health gain: adding years to life and life to years
- A mixed economy of statutory and independent activity in the health and social care field
- A move to a primary care-led NHS
- The need for better management and targeting of services
- Cost-effective and efficient services which are evidence-based and outcome-driven
- Encouraging and responding to the views of service users and potential users of services
- A focus on vulnerable people with lifetime mental ill-health
- Health promotion and prevention

As Tudor (1996) points out, there is no formal mental *health* policy from the state, instead the focus is upon mental *illness*. Furthermore, an emphasis on the needs of the severely mentally ill can exclude a broader population approach to mental health and its promotion. However, the themes described above have in turn been influenced by a range of social policy. Jones (1994), for example, describes the 1980s as a decade of considerable flux and reviews key changes, including welfare policy, employment and unemployment, social security, local government, housing, education, social services and social work. Thus, the potential for mental health as well as mental illness issues to be addressed directly and indirectly is wider than the NHS.

What does this mean to the potential mental health promotion practitioner?

The philosophy and cultural changes that have taken place within health and social care services have had and continue to have enormous repercussions for how mental ill-health is to be addressed towards the latter part of the twentieth century. Influences beyond psychiatry and the treatment and care of the mentally ill will shape a new set of arrangements and approaches. Within such policy can be seen the elements which are of significance for positive health and for its promotion.

Policy needs to be considered in the world within which it takes place. For example, the media and other interests, coupled with high-profile events in which psychiatric patients commit crimes or experience lack of care, have placed mental illness high on a range of agendas. This needs to be placed in the social and cultural context of concerns about crime and safety, morality and community *per se*. Whilst the policy focus has been on people with severe mental ill-health, the debate can and should be widened. The causation and amelioration as well as prevention and educational strategies can all be considered for this group and the population at large: a population which, thanks to health and social policy changes, can no longer rely on institutions to be separate worlds in which madness is controlled and contained. Citizens shocked, horrified or annoyed at the apparent lack or coordination of care and services have deep-rooted fears of madness in others and ultimately in themselves. As such they are also at the political forefront of existing and developing policy. The social 'raw nerve' that mental illness touches can allow a wider awareness and range of responses to mental ill-health. It provides opportunities to reflect upon our own health and to determine society's status in terms of the comprehensive care it does or does not provide to vulnerable citizens. It is at this juncture that we briefly examine mental illness policy.

Policy for mental illness

Butler (1993) describes a range of approaches to 'solving' the social problem of mental illness. From the post-war period these included the new welfare policies developed for health and social care, Care in the

Community, and finally a market economic policy (see Chapter 7). There has also been a gradual introduction of prevention, education and promotion of health which has developed in the area of mental health and mental illness (see Box 2.2).

Box 2.2 **'Solving' the problem of mental illness – a resumé of policy from the eighteenth century to the twentieth century (adapted from Butler 1993)**

1744–1845	Informal provision made by the local parish using the workhouse and the private madhouses
1845–1890	The building of the new public asylums
1890–1930	New lunacy laws introduced requiring the use of certification before admission to the asylums
1930–1948	The psychiatric and a medical model of mental illness increasingly accepted
1948–1954	New welfare policies developed for health and social care
1954–1975	Introduction and use of the new technology of drugs
1975–1990	Care in the Community forms the basis for public policy
1991 to date	The marketplace introduced as a shaper of health and social care with an increased emphasis on interagency cooperation. Needs-led service provision with user/carer input

---

We anticipate that a new phase is possible and desirable. This is a healthy public policy which draws upon the skills and expertise of a wider range of agencies and services than health and social care. Similar policy shifts can be identified in the fields of public health and of health promotion. The emergence of the public health movement, for example, can be traced to the late nineteenth century with a recognition, which still holds today, that prevention of ill-health and the promotion of health come about by social and environmental policy changes rather than by medical advances (Table 2.1).

Table 2.1
The range of public health activity and its focus from the late nineteenth century to the present

Activity	Focus
Late nineteenth century: Public Health Acts and Medical Officers of Health	Environment issues
Early twentieth century: Immunization, family planning	Personal preventive medicine
World War II: Hospital and treatment services	Medical and drug intervention
Today: Social and economic determinants of health	Healthy public policy

The policies and consequent resource allocation within which mental illness policy has moved can be traced in the same broad time spans (Table 2.2). Treatments, philosophy and practice of community care can also be seen to have followed a similar path. This demonstrates how such policy has moved from isolation, to control, cure and prevention.

Table 2.2
The range of mental health activity and its focus from the late nineteenth century to the present

Activity	Focus
Late nineteenth century: Building of asylums	Policy of containment and controlled environment
Early twentieth century: Immunization, family planning	Policy of personal preventive medicine: mental hygiene, eugenics
World War II: Hospital and treatment services	Medical and drug intervention; psychiatry in general medical hospital
Today: Community-focused services	Community Care: psychosocial interventions

The more contemporary policy and practice in mental health remains dominated by a value system torn between individual consumerism and social structural change. This is borne out in the tensions of mental health policy that is based upon degrees of social control while at the same time advocating policy for independence and empowerment.

Policy for care and treatment

Community Care

Since April 1991, the primary responsibility for planning, coordinating and paying for support services has been assigned to local authority social service departments. This significant policy change has placed an emphasis on work with the private sector to achieve cost-effective provision. The proposals were intended to lead to wider choice, control, accountability and a greater autonomy for users of services. The reality of non-hospital care has been problematic since the policy was introduced and adopted. The implementation of Caring for People (DOH 1989a) was delayed until April 1993 as local government raised concerns about how the new measures could be put in place.

Putting the community *per se* into its new role of carer has also not been a task that can be legislated for, nor has a policy been produced to make it work. A lack of preparation of the general community for this new role and the assumption that a caring and support infrastructure exists have resulted in friction between statutory bodies implementing government policy and local communities and communities of interest. It has been the service user who has borne the brunt of tenancy tensions on supported housing, planning applications for group homes and general misconceptions of mental ill-health and disability in general.

Ross *et al.* (1993) see the problems of Community Care (see Box 2.3) as being as much a part of the community itself as of professional mental health staff, especially in relation to prejudice and stigma. They identify as key issues: nonstigmatization, coping with crises, housing, employment and leisure, and day care. They stress the need to move away from looking at deficits all the time, which hides the strengths of users.

Box 2.3 **Aims of the Community Care Act (1990)**

- To end the confusion and fragmentation of responsibilities for the provision of services between social security, health, local authorities, private and voluntary provision
- To encourage private and voluntary provision
- To make services more accountable

The result of the policy implementation of Caring for People into Community Care has been to lose touch with original principles which placed great emphasis on choice and independent living. Perhaps as a consequence of professional territorialism, inadequate resource structure and an unknowing and unnerved general public, the opportunity for greater individual control has been replaced by case managers coordinating and managing care packages.

In its report into Community Care for People with Severe Mental Illness, the Mental Health Foundation (1994), for example, identifies commissioning arrangements as a way of influencing and shaping service delivery for this vulnerable group. These arrangements include health authorities, local authorities and fundholding practices. This collection of agencies and their combination are crucial if the policy of Community Care is to be achieved. The purchasing power of these agencies is also a result of various government policies formulated and adopted into management and work in the last decade in the United Kingdom. Indeed, such has been the extent of policy which has reformed the NHS and social services, many of the consequences of policy implementation are only now being tested and adapted into real settings.

There is more to policy which can influence health (and the promotion of mental health) than mental illness policy, and it is this that we shall now examine.

Community Care requires a network of services to be in place. How do you think this can be achieved?

What is the role of the non-mental-health specialist in Community Care?

Equity and health

Inequalities in health are a considerable challenge for public health policy. Without action for equity in health policy, treatment and care for mental illness is a limited exercise. Whitehead (1990) argues that equity and health are important owing to evidence that disadvantaged groups have higher morbidity, mortality and experience of illness. Another key reason is that 'Other dimensions of health and well-being show a similar pattern of blighted quality of life. In many countries unemployed people have poorer mental health' (p.3). Dahlgren and Whitehead (1992) recommend action on low income, unhealthy living conditions, working conditions, unemployment and personal lifestyle factors and action on restricted access to health care to reduce inequalities in health status. Factors influencing health include:

- Age, sex and heredity
- Individual lifestyle factors
- Social and community influences
- Living and working conditions
- General socioeconomic, cultural and environmental conditions

---

Social and economic context for health

The more the determinants of health are recognized and understood, the more inescapable is the conclusion that a person's health cannot be divorced from the social and economic environment in which they live.

(Benzeval *et al.* 1995)

A further review by Whitehead (1995) suggests four different levels for policy initiatives which can influence inequalities in health (Box 2.4). This international review of policy initiatives which have tackling inequalities as their focus is described below.

1. Strengthening individuals. This includes 'person-based strategies' supporting individuals' knowledge, motivation and skills to equip them to modify behaviour or deal with external health hazards. Example: Stress management or counselling for the unemployed to prevent mental illness. This is the area that most practitioners will focus their efforts upon.

2. Strengthening communities. This includes collective responses to external health hazards. This is achieved by maximizing the important role of family, friends, voluntary agencies and the community as a whole. The need for social cohesion and the need to create conditions for communities to work cooperatively are important here. Example:

Community development approaches to local defined health issues, such as racial harassment, crime or substance misuse. This is an area that practitioners are expected to support and encourage.

3. Improving access to essential facilities and services. Policies to establish the foundations for health including housing, clean water, health care, education and employment and training. Example: Public health advocacy through alliances to improve services and access to them. Practitioners here may be involved in a health alliance or through their professional or union bodies lobbying for policy changes.

4. Encouraging macroeconomic and cultural change. A whole-population approach to reducing inequality rather than individual, group or locality based. Example: Labour market policies such as the European minimum wage. This is the area the practitioner is least likely to influence directly.

Box 2.4 **Whitehead's four levels**

- Strengthening individuals
- Strengthening communities
- Improving access to essential facilities and services
- Encouraging macroeconomic and cultural change

How then can policy for health as well as health care and treatment be influenced?

Influencing policy

Ham (1992) describes the sources of 'policy inputs', that is factors which influence policy. These factors bring bargaining, negotiation and compromise into the development of health policy. They include:

- Pressure groups – awareness raising and lobbying
- The mass media – campaigning journalism
- NHS authorities – policy making as well as implementing
- Consultation systems – formal bodies such as the Health Advisory Service
- Government – ministers and civil servants

There is clearly room for the practitioner to influence policy development at all these levels. While the voluntary, user and carer lobby of policy makers has come to the fore, there is scope for the health promoter to support them in this role. And within professional and personal roles practitioners can support and encourage influences on policy in their own field: workplace policy on racism, equal opportunities, and

How far do you feel historical and contemporary policy has been driven by political and social forces. Is this desirable?

What do you see as the key policies for influencing mental illness service provision?

Are there policies which might benefit the population's mental health?

the development of policy to combat harassment and bullying. In the the wider arena, professional bodies can exert considerable influence on the formation and implementation of national and local policy as it affects practice. Being attuned to such possibilities is a key role for the mental health as well as the mental illness practitioner.

We will now go on to examine contemporary policy to identify aspects which are relevant to mental illness and to mental health and its promotion. Several areas of policy will be discussed. However, even the policy for mental illness care and treatment ensures that participation, intersectoral collaboration, critique and alternatives to state policy are more openly acknowledged and are in the process of finding their rightful place in mainstream psychiatry.

Policy and the public dimension

All health and social care policy in the mental illness and mental health field exerts influence to varying degrees upon all citizens. However, there are specific policies which attempt to address the general population. The role of public health policy will now be discussed.

Healthy public policy

Healthy cities: the Sheffield framework

The World Health Organization (WHO 1994) in a review of 49 Healthy City initiatives describes the participants in action for healthy cities as creating social change. Through a process of healthy public policy the role that a host of agencies and services have in improving and sustaining health can be developed. Such an approach can influence a range of policies at the social as well as health-related levels. While apparently far removed from health and social care policy, the city, town or any community has to absorb and adapt to a whole range of policy. The principles and practice of the Healthy City movement enable a broad range of policy to be coordinated at a strategic level and implemented more constructively. It also allows an opportunity to embrace a much wider vision of health and social care and responsibility. A broader definition and range of solutions can be considered, so making it of particular relevance for promoting the mental health of the general population.

In Sheffield as part of an extensive consultation exercise entitled 'Our City – Our Health' (Healthy Sheffield 1991) individuals, groups, communities and organizations identified factors which were seen to affect health and what action could be taken to improve it and to reduce inequalities in health in the city. The result has been the production of an action plan highlighting three key themes: poverty, discrimination and the environment. These themes are the foundation for tackling fourteen action areas ranging from accident prevention, carers' health and housing to education, violence and aggression. Mental and emotional well-being is one element in a Framework for Action to improve the health of a city.

Objective of Framework for Action

To set an agenda for multiagency work to improve people's health and to shape the conditions which have an effect on health. The development of this agenda and the detailed work to deliver it will be a long-term process taking place over the coming years. It will require continued and joint work across agencies and in partnership with the many communities in the city. (Snell 1994)

Unlike much of the formal health and social care strategy and policy, this reflects the noninstitutional and nonmedical components which are required to promote health. It is reproduced here to highlight the differences and to some degree the similarities of policy and possible practice activity as set out in more mental illness-focused material. The relevance of a broad public health and health promotion effect has been developed elsewhere. Dalgard *et al.* (1991) for example, examined mental health from a systems perspective. They cite the practice in Nova Scotia which aimed to promote the mental health of a population with a high level of mental illness. This was achieved by increasing social integration through social support and mutual aid, improving educational opportunities and increasing economic resources. The decade after these recommendations were implemented saw a reduction in the prevalence of mental illness. In describing strategies and policies for promoting mental health, they highlight as important political and legal measures and direct community work by mental health workers.

They also cite the example of neighbourhood planning guidelines for Oslo, which include multigenerational communities, varying housing types and involvement of local tenants in the planning process. This emphasis on the importance of wider factors influencing the prevalence of mental health and mental illness is in contrast to some of the more individual-focused measures proposed as part of traditional policy. As was highlighted in the examination of the Mental Health Nursing Review, the boundaries need to shift from good-quality patient care to wider, whole-community responses to treatment, care and promotion of mental health. The Framework for Action approach adopted in

Sheffield demonstrates the need to take a much wider view on mental health and illness than the individual actually or potentially requiring support or care. Other examples of a Healthy City approach with a mental health perspective are identified in a review by WHO (1994):

- **Glasgow women's health policy:** A healthy public policy has been developed including the views of a range of women in voluntary groups. This process has identified needs not met by existing services such as mental health problems related to the role of women in society. (Case study 4. WHO 1994)
- **Self-help centres for teachers in Vienna:** This is seen as recognizing health promotion works by developing personal skills in a supportive environment. This project set up a service to meet stress in teachers by providing a centre for anonymous help. Self-help and therapy sessions are also part of the initiative. (Case study 9. WHO 1994)

Health and social care policy and the professions

Mental health promotion and the Butterworth report

The publication of the report of the Mental Health Nursing Review Team 'Working in Partnership: a Collaborative Approach to Care' (Butterworth 1994) was the first since 1968. Chaired by Professor Butterworth, its terms of reference were to identify the future requirements for skilled nursing care in the light of developments in the provision of services for people with mental illness. This included a re-examination of all aspects of its policy and practice. The Review makes a total of 42 recommendations in six key areas:

1. Building relationships with service users
2. The practice of nursing
3. The delivery of services
4. Issues that are challenging
5. Research in mental health nursing
6. Pre- and post-registered education.

The recommendations range from a focus of attention on the needs of people with an enduring mental illness to the importance of providing information to service users and carers. It highlights new roles for mental health nurses, including psychosocial interventions and liaison nursing with general medical and primary care services. A suggested framework for collaborative working by nurses, midwives and health visitors in mental health care is proposed which constitutes a preventative model to reduce the incidence of mental illness by working with vulnerable groups and developing early detection and interventions approaches.

The Review recognizes that the increase in GP fundholding will result in an increase in demand for mental health nurses. Equally, Community Care initiatives mean that people with enduring mental health problems are coming under the wing of primary care. In order for these people's physical as well as mental health needs to be met, mental health nurses need to act as a consistent point of contact for users, carers and other professionals. As part of the Care Programme Approach, mental health nurses act as key workers to coordinate packages of care for users admitted to hospital and those about to be discharged. Therefore, their role, especially with the primary health care team, is crucial in both the planning and delivery of health and social care. Five areas of policy are recognized to be relevant to the future work of mental health nurses:

1. The NHS commissioning and provider system
2. The NHS and Community Care Act (DOH 1990)
3. The Children Act (1989)
4. The Patients' Charter (DOH 1991)
5. The Health of the Nation (DOH 1992a, 1993a, 1994a).

The Butterworth report (Butterworth 1994) also describes a 'policy push', referring to research with a focus on the delivery of health care as cited in documents which emphasize the nursing contribution to research such as the Health of the Nation – Key Area Handbook: Mental Illness (DOH 1993a).

What then are the critical elements of the review and their implications for the practitioner promoting mental health? In the executive summary (p.5) it states: 'As approaches to care become increasingly centred on the individual, the mental health nurse's contribution – with its emphasis on interpersonal relationships and operational flexibility – will be critical to success.' It goes on to emphasize that the principle of choice for service users and carers should be at the foundation for practitioners. And it stresses the importance of the relationship they have with such practitioners and the service they represent. The report highlights models of good mental health nursing which have the following features:

- Client assessment involving clients and their carers
- An understanding of the needs and perceptions of the local community and positive efforts to promote awareness
- A conscious effort to deal sensitively with issues of race, creed and gender

This is very much a health-promoting focus. These models encourage the practitioner to take account of active participation by involving the client and significant others in key decision making to enable choice and information sharing and by a recognition of 'felt needs' – the issues, concerns and experience of local communities – and actively raising awareness of mental ill-health. There are two methods available to make these three features operate successfully. A traditional method employs existing structures and systems and implements policy. An MHP methodology acknowledges that, in the area of acute mental health services, such traditional elements are in some respects

Table 2.3
Standard and MHP methods of working with mental health issues

Feature	Traditional method	MHP method
Assessment involving the clients and their carers	Invitation to meetings	Involvement of advocacy services
	Professional leadership and focus	Support of user-focused approaches
	Literature produced by professionals	Development of information by and for users/carers
An understanding of the needs and perceptions of the local community and positive efforts to promote awareness	Mapping out of the high-profile groups and organizations	Mapping out of all mental health stakeholders
	Public meetings	Focus groups
	Professional/voluntary forums	Community-led assessment of needs, recommendations and solutions
	Literature produced by professionals	Community inspired/ produced resources
A conscious effort to deal sensitively with issues of race, creed and gender	Training for staff on culture and race	Anti-oppressive training for all staff
	Equal opportunity policy	Proactive attempts to involve marginalized individuals and communities in methods described above
	Use of interpretation and translation services	Encouragement of support groups for minority ethnic users

fashioned around a medical and legislative framework. However, the boundaries are pushed out to consider self-empowerment and collective action for mental health. This is demonstrated in Table 2.3 in which the three features identified by the Review are placed against the existing and potential methods of responding to assessment, public perceptions and power relations.

What this demonstrates is that the shift from standard to mental health-promoting methods of working does not require considerable investment in resources. There are evident training experiences and exposure to different styles and culture of operation required, but on the whole these can be achieved within current activity. It is about putting into practice the nurturing and enabling role that is part of good mental health practice. Service providers in collaboration with the purchasers of their services and the client group itself need to negotiate the extent and feasibility of supporting such methods.

The Review poses many questions and leaves at the door of the profession a whole series of considerations. In the context of other policy change and implementation in the mental health field, the specialist nurse has considerable opportunity to exert influence on policy implementation. In this way policy can be as much about mental health promotion as mental illness care and prevention.

Nursing and public health issues

Making it Happen (DOH 1995b) was a re-examination of professional issues for nurses, midwives and health visitors as part of the NHS reforms. Several elements which nursing as a professional group can influence were highlighted, including health policy. The report makes a total of thirteen recommendations to purchasers, research and other professional and national bodies (see Box 2.5).

There is scope for nurses to become involved in social, organizational and policy work in practice. This can include active participation in the implementation of public health policy, involvement in research and educational strategies, and a recognition of European policies as they affect health. The contribution of health visiting in the field of public health and of influencing policies affecting health is given prominence in the report. As was evident in the mental health nursing review, the relationship between specialist mental health nursing and their counterparts in primary care settings such as health visitors, district and practice nurses allows options for collaborative work at the health policy as well as the health care levels. The combined strength of nursing to identify and highlight need is vital for the public, purchasers and

---

Why is the approach to care becoming more centred on the individual? Is this research based or a response to government policy and an individualistic approach to mental health care?

The principle of choice also allows people to choose alternatives to mental health interventions practised by nurses. What is their role in examining alternatives?

Does the relationship nurses have with service users go beyond the individual to the family, work colleagues and the community at large?

Box 2.5 **Features of a public health approach to nursing**

- A knowledge of whole-population health needs. A population consists of identified client groups, whole communities or large geographical areas
- An emphasis on collective and collaborative action
- A recognition of people as members of groups, not only as individuals
- A public health perspective which anchors clinical and nonclinical care in the social, organizational and policy aspects of health development
- A focus on health promotion, in enabling people to increase control over and improve their health, combined with preventing disease

Making it Happen (DOH 1995b)

policy makers alike. And, as demonstrated in a Healthy City approach, it enables a broader view and involvement of health professionals to 'cross reference' health issues and plan action accordingly.

Public health nursing

Public health in nursing, midwifery and health visiting practice is about commissioning health services and providing professional care through organized collaboration in the NHS and society, to protect and promote health and well-being, prolong life and prevent ill-health in local communities, groups and populations.

Making it Happen (DOH 1995b, p.5)

A resumé of the recommendations and their focus can enable several aspects of public health nursing to be considered. There is a considerable range of nurse practice at the hospital, community and intervening levels – a pool of talent and expertise to draw upon. There are also opportunities as part of the raft of policy shifts in health and social care to scrutinize role, function and activity. And internurse, interagency and community-focused collaboration can implement national and local policy in a more meaningful and creative way. If it is delivered within a framework of community participation and community development, the possibilities are enormous.

The Royal College of Nursing (1993, pp.11–13) suggests a focus on training in primary care and with GPs including a 'vigorous education programme for primary health care teams on handling anxiety and depression'.

The consequences of changes resulting from current health and social policy are not fully known. The development of local primary care purchasing in which the general practitioner can make wider decisions on which services and resources to purchase for his or her practice population have implications for nursing. A tension may arise between the professional and policy demands of local purchasing, a Healthy City approach, professional development, and policy for practice demanded by the NHS Executive. This also has resonance from a policy perspective in terms of the recently published *Variations in Health* paper (DOH 1995c) which acknowledges that public education programmes, for example, that do not have continuing support will not flourish. This has implications, too, for primary health care work which is dictated at a purchasing level around annual negotiations and also other sources of funding which are time limited. Decision making may be swayed as much by judgements, values and misconceptions of professionals and the services they *can* and *could* provide as by illness needs and community health needs. If it is the latter, then the only route is a social model of health, and therefore health-promoting practice is inevitable. There is a role in policy development and interpretation of policy for this coalition of nursing practitioners and managers.

A key policy change has been the division of health authorities and hospital and community services as part of the purchaser/provider division of NHS managerial responsibility. This will be discussed in more detail in Chapter 7. A key element in the policy changes around health care planning and provision in the mental health field that has also been significantly influenced is the overall policy commitment to a primary care-led NHS.

Primary care

The importance of primary care for MHP is threefold. At a service level it is the key point of contact for people in distress who may require a range of specialist assessment and assistance via referral mechanisms. At another level it is closer to where mental health services see their location as teams operate from a community focus. And at another level the potential for a broader definition and practice of primary health care widens the scope of practice and interagency influence on practice populations. This also affects clusters of practices, to improve the health of communities as well as to prevent, treat and refer on people's ill-health needs.

Primary care is also pivotal in the policy changes that have swept the NHS and is crucial to the redeployment of services, skills and activity in the mental health field. As the Alma Ata (WHO 1978) definition

How would you improve the public's health and what policy would you consider most relevant to do this?

What are the strengths and weaknesses of a more active public health role for nursing?

Can a hospital be healthy, and if so how can it promote mental health?

Primary health care: a definition

Primary health care is essential health care made universally accessible to individuals and families in the community by means acceptable to them, through their full participation and at a cost that the community and country can afford. It forms an integral part of both the country's health system of which it is the nucleus and of the overall social and economic development of the community.

Declaration in Alma Alta (WHO 1978)

highlights, this also allows opportunities to support community participation and health alliances and to address health inequalities.

Why is primary care important for MHP?

- Its location – within communities and located close to other community infrastructure.
- Its function – as a setting for health and other care services and in access to specialized treatment
- Its variety – provision of social, preventive and educational aspects

In October 1995 a debate was initiated on primary care by the Secretary of State for Health. A document, *Primary Care: The Future* (DOH 1996a), has resulted and consists of a collection of the views of patients, professionals and managers on how primary care should be developed. A list of what primary care should provide is given in Chapter 10, and significantly it includes addressing the health needs of local communities as well as individuals. This is a potentially broader vision of primary care and one which ties in with an MHP approach in terms of participatory approaches and methods which value and utilize the skills and resource base of communities themselves. However, the report rather narrowly defines patient and carer information and involvement as 'developing choice and information but also recognizing patient responsibilities as well as rights' (p.7). While we would not disagree that accountability lies with individuals as well as professionals, it is difficult to exercise responsibility without adequate resources and support. The report stresses that a range of options will be considered to make working arrangements and contracts for primary care practitioners flexible. The reality, however, is that they will only consider piloting of options such as salaried GPs employed by NHS trusts, a definition of core general medical services (GMS), practice-based contracts and extended fundholding.

Primary health care services

Given that more is expected of primary care – and in the mental illness field this is evident as the structures and systems that once cared for people's long- and medium-term mental health needs no longer exist – there is concern that there has not been a commensurate shift in resources from secondary to primary care. Coupled with perceptions of an erosion of professional autonomy on the part of clinicians there is distinct tension as well as opportunity within primary health care.

The policy context for an increasing interest in and focus on primary health care has been influenced by various items of implicit and explicit policy: the Local Voices initiative, Health for All, a move towards organizational decentralization in private and public sectors. In terms of primary care we have moved from a locality planning and management model in the 1970s and 1980s, with local collaboration, bottom-up planning and limited budget devolution, to a more contemporary locality purchasing model in the wake of fundholding, a variety of forms and few examples of mainstream budget decentralization.

Do you agree with a broad definition of primary health care? How can this be taken forward into practical action?

In what ways could you use the focus of primary care to address health inequality?

Government MHP Policy: Health of the Nation

The Health of the Nation (1992a) is part of a health policy which has placed the onus on services and practitioners to improve upon and change how they manage and deliver services, including mental health. It reflects the WHO aim of setting out national and local targets and providing a comprehensive strategy and policy approach to health. The goal of Health of the Nation is to secure continuing improvement in the general health of the population. It identifies five key areas for particular attention including 'mental illness'.

Each Key Area has objectives and targets and there is considerable scope for a range of health promotion models and methods to meet them. There are also common issues for mental health and the other key areas, for example stress, coping, loss and control. The emotional impact of ill-health *per se* and the emotions that surround our health and well-being are such that all the Key Areas could be said to have our psychological state at their core. The demands of services for work within this and other health-related policy have at their root changes in thinking and in behaviour. It is for this reason that the mental (the emotional, feelings) aspect of health runs through all of the Key Areas. This common foundation establishes possibilities for the practitioner to highlight the mental health as well as the mental illness aspects of a range of health issues. The National Targets for Mental Illness confine themselves to measurable aspects of contemporary mental health services. While not ideal, they present a useful starting point to consider creative ways in which they could be achieved. It is this flexibility of interpretation of government policy in order to achieve the goals that provides an opportunity for mental health promotion. Coupled with the emphasis of user involvement in the community care process, the five policies that the Nursing Review identifies, and cross referencing of other action areas outlined by Healthy Sheffield (1991), there is scope for a range of interventions and activity that do not have to be constrained by adherence to a single policy for the practitioner. In fact, part of a MHP malaise may be the result of almost too much policy and its interrelationships. This is why the practitioner needs to understand this range and identify those elements they are expected to react to and those around which they can be more proactive.

The national mental health charity MIND has produced a policy statement on Health of the Nation (MIND 1994a). It calls for joint work with a range of agencies in order to develop new local targets with a stronger user focus. MIND also identifies possible problems associated with the existing targets such as a shift to more oppressive practices. It offers a number of new targets including those relating to service access, antidiscrimination legislation, positive mental health awareness in schools and tackling inequalities in social security policy.

One of the limitations of the Health of the Nation is that the National Health Service predominates. At a policy and strategy level it is easy for other key disciplines within the mental health field, most notably social services, to see the contribution to the targets as a health service responsibility and obligation. The references to health alliances and partnership are irrelevant if there is no common ownership as to the achievement of the strategy. Implementation could be seen to occur by default or as resting on the infrastructure of the NHS. From a health-promoting and health policy perspective this is a narrow view. In many senses the role of the mental health promoter should then be about raising this issue, identifying where responsibilities are joint and ensuring that all agencies take on board the mental health message regardless of historical approaches to mental health service planning and policy and provision of services.

What is at stake is a need for policy to improve health care and treatment services, to make them more relevant and less oppressive to those who use them or are contemplating using them. We also need healthy public policy to address the needs of the 'inherently at risk' – those vulnerable citizens who require support and a support infrastructure. The community itself needs to become mentally healthy in order to achieve this. Action on poverty, discrimination and the environment are all required here. Health and social care practitioners cannot be expected to alter society radically. The limitations of their professional codes and practices prevent such a change in direction. However, what is possible is a cultural shift and a more sceptical reading of policy and its implications. Policy begets policy and this effect can result in objectives and values, established as part of an initial change in practice, not being implemented as intended. It is the role of the practitioner to see that objectives and values which underpin public health are sustained and championed.

Professionals are the group who operationalize governmental policy from national to the local implementation level. They act as gatekeepers and referring agents, not just to service provision, but they also hold a range of local interpretations, professionally and organizationally, of such policy. They can reformulate and interpret in innovative, obstructive or destructive ways. They also have a tension between what they personally and professionally may feel in terms of the new priorities and the management structures that they have to operate within.

Conclusion

From the current raft of material produced in the mental health field we identify a range of themes which run through all the documents. For some there is an interchangeable terminology of 'alliances', 'networks' and 'collaboration'. This demonstrates the success of infiltration into mainstream policy and review by alternative or even radical thinking. However, the terminology – the language of mental health promotion – is easily adopted by policy, strategy and operational activity by psychiatry. This is to be welcomed and encouraged, although with adoption comes responsibility. To take on board the message is not enough. The full implications require organizations and services to reflect on existing processes and practice which may require fundamental shifts in attitude and activity. This is the biggest challenge for services and their practitioners to face up to. The next chapter draws attention to these key developments in relation to their significance for mental health promotion and community participation for MHP.

Practice checklist

- Appreciate the relevance for policy shifts for practice — look critically at their origins and impact.

- Utilize policy for the benefit of MHP — maximize opportunities for influencing policy.

- Become aware of local policy for the workplace on harassment, antiracism, mental health.

- Look critically at social and welfare policy and its relevance for health and mental health.

Community participation and involvement

3

Health for All is, as a matter of principle, a movement for people. They have the right to equal opportunity in health, the right to health care, the right to be informed, and the right to be involved as partners in decision-making and action affecting their health. Partnership for health means the encouragement of intersectoral collaboration and multisectoral action and the promotion of community participation. (WHO 1991, p.66)

Key themes:

- Community participation and involvement
- Health alliances and professional service providers
- Health alliances as defined and determined by the policy/strategy makers

Overview

This chapter examines the issue of community participation at three levels:

1. **Community participation and involvement:** the significance of this for genuine power sharing and shaping of the health and social care agendas to take into account nonprofessional views. Important within this discussion is the role that professionals themselves can play in order to assist, enable and encourage vulnerable groups and the mentally ill and their carers take part in this process. A checklist to think through some of the key issues around consultation is presented

2. **Health alliances and the professional worker:** the example of mental health service users is discussed, and possible ways of becoming involved in a health alliance approach

3. **Health alliances as defined and determined by the policy/strategy makers:** here the example overlaps with level 2 in terms of how, for example, nurses are expected to operationalize the statements and documents produced via the Health of the Nation.

We will begin our discussion by an examination of definitions of community participation and what community involvement might look like for the mental health promoter.

Introduction

Health alliances are integral to the role of the health practitioner as mental health promoter. Whether in statutory, voluntary or user organizations, such alliances enable practitioners to become the messenger, mediator and critic of government health policy. For citizens and communities it can be an enabling function allowing a proactive response to factors and influences on mental and emotional health. How far this can extend to empowerment remains to be seen, but the benefits of developing and sustaining networks on mental health issues are attractive. This role of brokerage by practitioners between health policy and the public they serve allows a unique opportunity to maximize a wealth of skills and experiences of service users and carers to shape the health agenda. It also requires honesty and commitment from the statutory agencies, as this powerful position can also culminate in tokenism or a lack of clarity. Not only is the process a potentially creative or destructive one, but we start without a common definition. As Naidoo and Wills (1994) point out there are significant differences in the terms used to describe health alliances, including:

- Multiagency
- Intersectoral
- Inter- or multidisciplinary working
- Joint planning and teams

The various services and agencies relate and define themselves within these terms and this, in turn, may have consequences for how they respond and react within a health alliance framework. The community mental health team, for example, will be both familiar and comfortable with operating in a multidisciplinary role. This may prove problematic if a more open approach is required when working with, for example, local mental health user groups. In this context the collective protection of multiple disciplines may be interpreted as psychiatric protectionism of the professional mental health agencies. The terms and definitions used in relation to health alliances require a degree of thought to be given before they are employed and a consensus to be reached. 'Health alliances' is a popular term within the health service in its purchasing and providing functions. However, 'intersectoral collaboration', which has its origins in the WHO global strategy Health for All relates more to joint working across sector boundaries, including industry, business, commerce, statutory and voluntary organizations and community groups. Given its Health for All origins, it is a terminology that we need to consider reapplying.

There is also a negative aspect to the networking and collaborative intelligence gathering which are ingredients of a health alliance approach. It is important for purchasers and providers of services to reflect public opinion and to ensure that services are of a high quality; inadequate consultation masquerading as intersectoral collaboration can infuriate and demotivate the public. To explore these issues further this chapter examines three elements of healthy alliances.

1. Issues of community participation and involvement

Community participation is of paramount importance to the area of health alliances and collaborative practice. A health alliance can be a response to a health issue and such a response does not have to be expert driven or coordinated by a professional discipline. There is room for individuals, groups and communities to mobilize on single or multiple health concerns and realize possible solutions to those concerns. This involves drawing on a range of views, opinions and support from a whole host of groups and organizations. In the mental health field this could include:

- Local authority housing departments
- Local media
- Welfare rights services
- Day centres
- The Church
- Community and self-help groups
- Users and carers

Such network development may take precedence over the established disciplines of social work, primary care and specialist mental health workers from hospitals and community mental health teams. This can result in a range of views on a range of mental health themes: a broad umbrella of experience and expertise brought to bear on a particular issue. The very nature of a health alliance is that it moves away from the narrow confines of health as purely an illness matter and places it in its social context, making community participation an inevitable and welcome product of a genuine health alliance approach. However, it may be misinterpreted by statutory agencies as consultation on already formulated strategies. This differs from participation, which is about involving the community earlier in the process and about the community identifying its own needs. Smithies *et al.* (1990) describe the community participation movement as having three basic Health for All principles:

- Increasing community participation

- Encouraging more collaboration between statutory and voluntary sectors
- Highlighting and reducing inequalities in health

They elaborate these principles by providing a range of definitions of participation in the framework outlined in Table 3.1. Such an approach has implications particularly in relation to practice, effectiveness and evaluation. It is worth quoting Smithies *et al.* (1990) in more detail as to the implications of such an approach:

> This way of working can seem time-consuming and creates challenges for evaluation strategies. However, we believe that the process involved is as valuable as the outcome. The process is developmental, and as such work may progress into areas and activities that were not originally envisaged. This means that all parties need to be flexible and open to change, basing their work on commonly agreed principles rather than rigid goals. There is no doubt that many in positions of power will find this way of working alien. However, opportunities to work in new and innovative ways provide benefits for communities, bureaucrats and professionals alike.

Table 3.1 **Definitions of participation**			
	Formal participation	High or low participation in policy making, planning, etc.	Publicity about hospital closure, inviting comments, representatives, community forums
	Community action	Activity or process undertaken that involves action to obtain change	Pressure groups, advocacy projects, lobbying, direct action
	Facilitating processes	Community organization, enabling practices and related skills	Community analysis, neighbourhood planning, developing skills
	Professional and community interface	People, communities and professional dialogue	Training for community workers, joint forums, participation groups, organizational development
	Strategic support	Initiatives/policies which support community action	Funding, training, research, information

(Smithies *et al.* 1990, Section 4: Summary p.61)

Several comments can be made on this statement. The first is its historical context. The reforms of the NHS and social services are now such that the whole area of outcomes and health gain has gained prominence. This needs to be considered in relation to evaluation strategies, targeting of community intervention and review mechanisms in the area of community participation, health alliances and MHP. Secondly, if we are to talk of promoting mental health as including those citizens and communities that do not fall within the definition of formal psychiatric diagnosis, but whose individual or collective health and well-being are threatened or compromised, then we need to consider that a range of participation processes such as those on community safety, housing, environment, welfare and nutrition will all have mental health benefits. These are beyond the immediate control and influence of the mainstream mental health service providers. It is important, therefore, in the early stages of health alliance development to identify and clarify these elements and draw themes of mental health from existing programmes and interventions. This can allow agenda setting by viewing mental health in a social context. The consequences of professionals and communities working cooperatively to improve not just the physical structures of neighbourhoods, communities and the people who live and work in them but also the emotional and mental benefits which flow from such an approach are enormous. As Healthy Sheffield (1993) points out in a strategy for community development and health, there are various degrees of participation and 'Genuine community participation can only be developed when support and resources have been made available and enabling structures have been fostered over a period of time.' (p.18). This can best be demonstrated using the model of Brager and Specht (1973). This sets out a linear sequence of participation ranging from high to low participation with intervening levels of consultation and advice. It is set out in Table 3.2.

Degree of participation	Participants' action	Illustrative model	
Low	None	The community is told nothing.	Table 3.2 **Degree of participation**
	Receives information	The organization makes a plan and announces it. The community is convened for informational purposes; compliance is expected.	
	Is consulted	The organization tries to promote a plan and develop the support to facilitate acceptance of,	*(continued overleaf)*

Table 3.2 **Degree of participation** (*continued*)	**Degree of participation**	**Participants' action**	**Illustrative model**
			or give sufficient sanction to, the plan so that administrative compliance can be expected.
		Advises	The organization presents a plan and invites questions. It is prepared to modify the plan only if absolutely necessary.
		Plans jointly	The organization presents a tentative plan subject to change and invites recommendations from those affected.
		Has delegated authority	The organization identifies and presents a problem in to the community, defines the limits and asks the community to make a series of decisions which can be embodied in a plan which it will accept.
	High	Has control	The organization asks the community to identify the problems and to make all the key decisions regarding goals and means. It is willing to help the community at each step accomplish its own goals, even to the extent of administrative control of the programme.

For a level of participation that ties in with a mental health-promoting approach, we should be looking towards a high degree of involvement in which individuals and communities own and take control of the consultation process. A key concept is that of the organization assisting the community to accomplish this. If empowerment is to have any practical function in the real world then it has to include support, power sharing and an acknowledgement of the skills and expertise contained within communities themselves. This is also true of communities within hospital settings and other care settings. The end product for the formal agencies engaged in such an endeavour is not only that the quality, quantity and depth of the consultation and information will be better, but the process itself will have many positive outcomes. Being taken seriously and having to listen, negotiate and ask fundamental questions all constitutes valuable learning for organizations and communities alike. Also, given that a sense of control and of worth is a key foundation for good mental and emotional well-being, good consultation can be mental health-promoting. It is an essential element of the NHS reforms that local people – as consumers, actual or potential – should be able to have a say in service planning and development. This is an area of opportunity for the skills of community-based staff to key into such participation strategies and encourage and support the active involvement of the particular population groups they may work with. Labyrinth Training have been involved in a range of Local Voices initiatives and community development training. They have developed a framework of what should be included within a community involvement strategy. Such a framework for addressing community involvement highlights the importance of involving people in health and social care developments. It can also assist the varying professional elements within health and social care systems to locate where their skills and deficits may lie as part of such a process. Parts of the community involvement mechanisms in the past have rested on two false assumptions. Firstly, an assumption of the existence of a community and second, an assumption about the skills and methods of the professional in engaging with communities. The checklist described in Box 3.1 should ensure that skills, training, communication, methodology and equal-opportunity principles and practice are an integral part of such activity.

Box 3.1 **What needs to be in a community involvement strategy?**

Rationale: Why are we doing this? Is it for the health authority plans or purchasing intentions or is it to rethink how services are purchased?
Goals: What do we want to achieve?
Definitions: What is meant by 'involvement', 'local people', etc.
Equal opportunities: What role will this play in the work?
Policy: How does the involvement of local people link to other priorities?
Organization development: Is the organization ready for dealing with inputs and involvement from local people? What are the potential change implications for the organization? How can these be 'managed'?

Training: What are the skills and knowledge implications for staff? How might these be met?

Planning mechanisms: How might ideas, needs, concerns expressed by local people, user groups, etc. feed into planning cycles? Do they need to be adapted or changed?

Communication: How will information be shared around the organization, with the public, and with other agencies?

Methodology: What approaches might be used to involve people? What are the timescale and resource implications? What are the implications for skills?

Resource implications: What are the implications for staff time and priorities, finance, other resources such as computers, publishing? Who will coordinate the work?

Evaluation and monitoring: How will the work and its implications for change be monitored and evaluated? How will the effectiveness of different approaches be compared?

We suggest that this route to an understanding of the role of professionals involving communities is one that they should all undertake. The process itself and the lessons learned will be invaluable experience for any mental health-promoting work within a health alliance framework.

2. Health alliances and professional service providers

The health policy of the state is clear in its willingness to improve public participation. In 1992 *Local Voices* (DOH 1992b) was published and set out the rationale and examples of practice for health authorities to implement. Contemporary planning guidance also emphasizes the importance of public participation, particularly for service users and carers. As 'champions of the people' the health authorities are in a position to utilize existing resources, networks, terms of reference and research to undertake thorough and meaningful participation strategies that mean as much to the public as they do to the health professionals and governmental ideology. Such public involvement also allows for a broader debate about health issues. Donaldson (1995) sets out some practical steps which the professional could consider in relation to user consultation (see Box 3.2).

Genuine community participation and involvement within a health alliance framework will reflect on the limitations as well as the scope of mental health practitioners' experiences and knowledge base. In this way practitioners will begin to develop practice which is mental

Box 3.2 **User consultation**

- An organization-wide strategy for involving patients and carers as individuals, and as groups
- A long-term plan that enables trust and an infrastructure to be built up
- Training and support for staff at all levels of the organization, recognizing that it is a long-term learning process for health service staff and users
- Dedicated NHS staff to develop projects and links with the community
- Resources for community groups to develop their experience and skills
- Built-in evaluation from the start

(Donaldson 1995)

health-promoting. The journey to this conclusion requires critical analysis. Professionals within the mental health field have tended to see user involvement as ameliorating the distress of mental ill-health by the very process of involvement. In short, participation in whatever capacity is deemed to be 'therapeutic' and preventive. There remain problems with this assumption, the roots of which can be traced to the professional role of facilitation within a theory of empowerment. Stark (1986), for example, argues that preventive action should be discussed in terms of 'interventive pragmatism' and identifies several underlying conceptualizations which can be uncovered by an analysis of interventions:

- A public health model that is individually based
- A mental health education model which, combined with the public health model, remains concerned with the individual
- A social and community interventions model

In this, Stark argues that most professionals tend to carry their 'clinical view' into the field of prevention. 'Trying to maintain their status and competence as professionals and experts, they transfer the principles of their clinical education and experience to a very different setting. This person-oriented approach is definitely currently supported by a conservative social policy' (p.182). He argues that a preventive theory should be about social structure as well as individual and social behaviour. To achieve this mental health professionals need to understand fully the communities within which they work. This requires them to 'accept citizens in their own social environment' (p.183). Given that the notion of control is central to emotional and psychological well-being (Fernando 1993), this suggests that enhancement of the rights and needs of people or community groups is required – prevention of mental distress and promotion of mental health should be about building on strengths and abilities rather than on deficits and risks. It is also implied that to do this requires dialogue for a clear exchange of ideas, ideologies and opinions. This places the health and social care professionals in a potential dilemma. Are they the allies, enablers or bystanders in a participation culture? Professionals have the expertise, resources and opportunities to explore a range of options and approaches unavailable to users (Wilson 1995). There also remains the problem of health professionals acting as advocates on behalf of service users, when the professional's role is unclear (Gates 1995).

3. Primary care

A key setting for involving service users is in primary care. Recent discussion on the role of the nurse in this setting and activity is worth consideration in any exploration of participation strategies and health alliances. The terms of reference for the report *Nursing in Primary Health Care: New World, New Opportunities* (DOH 1993b) were to consider nursing services in the context of primary health care, and to recommend to ministers the steps necessary to ensure their effective development in both the short and the medium term. The report is bold in its introduction, stating: 'Primary health care in England is at the forefront of a health service revolution.' Primary health care is described as having two objectives: (1) to improve individual and family health; and (2) to improve health for total populations.

Within the context of the National Strategy, the Patients' Charter and Caring for People, the following point is made: 'The Health of the Nation reflects the political commitment to better health in which primary care services will play a key part, not least by involving individuals and communities in the maintenance and development of their own health' (p.3). The nurse's contribution in this is seen as flexibility and role clarification as well as improved interprofessional partnerships including voluntary agencies. This suggests that the government sees a dual role for these staff. It can be interpreted as a broad community development approach employing a health alliance approach. It cites the WHO definition of primary care and point 1.6 states: 'Primary health care is at its most effective when integrated with other health care services – including, of course, hospitals – and when it works in close collaboration with local social, welfare, environmental, and education systems – for example, through "healthy alliance".'

What are the benefits of a health alliance? Funnell *et al.* (1995) identify health alliances as arrangements for joint working, collaboration and cooperation between district health authorities and other agencies in order to work towards the achievement of Health of the Nation targets. This is clearly a narrower definition of health alliances than a Health for All one, although elements of it can be seen in the list of the benefits of a health alliance approach produced in government documentation. This list includes:

- More effective use of resources
- Broadening responsibility for health
- Breaking down barriers/improving knowledge
- Exchange of information
- Developing local health strategies
- Generating networks
- Developing seamless services

The explicit references to genuine collaborative practice utilizing the *process potential* of the health practitioner is significant for our discussion. In terms of the role of the nurse, 'development work', 'networks' and a broader view of health and the factors which can promote it are key to assisting user participation in the context of health alliances. Within the primary care setting there are opportunities for participation; the example of a patient participation group is described in Box 3.3.

Box 3.3 **Case example – primary care**

Partnership with patients. A practical guide to starting a patient participation group (Pritchard 1993)

This is a booklet aimed to help GPs, practice staff and patients to understand more about participation groups and how to initiate and sustain one. 'The major goal of patient participation is to help individuals to become involved in the organization of primary health care so that their needs are met more effectively' (p.3). Pritchard sets out eight areas of activity which such groups share:

1. Ensuring that goals are compatible
2. Seeking patient's views on services
3. Helping 'under-served' groups
4. Linking health care with other networks
5. A forum for suggestions and complaints
6. Promoting prevention and healthy lifestyle
7. Influencing other organizations
8. Supporting the work of the practice.

In a health policy environment of a primary care-led NHS and devolution of responsibility and budgets to the local level with fundholding and 'total purchasing', the role of the GP and accompanying team will require continued involvement in and refinement of interagency working and initiation of participation strategies.

Health policy and health alliances

Health of the Nation – Key Area Handbook: Mental Illness (DOH 1993a)

In Chapter 5, 'Developing Local Alliances', the action summary addressed to all NHS and SSD managers states:

> Develop better cooperative working between primary and secondary health care and between health and social services.

> Develop alliances with a wide range of other local and national organizations to develop mental health initiatives.

In the context of MHP the second element is the most relevant to consider as such mental health initiatives can potentially go beyond the confines of mental illness service provision.

The chapter acknowledges that the development of health alliances requires time, effort and understanding. However, this investment can result in

- More comprehensive collection and sharing of information on the local health picture
- Other agencies setting their own targets for mental health
- Coordinating action to maximize the effective use of resources, for example community care programmes
- A better understanding of mental illness and the contribution of social factors and alcohol and drug abuse to mental illness and suicide rates
- A better range of services for mentally disordered offenders, helping to avoid unnecessary imprisonment with the consequent risk of suicide or self-harm

The key alliances as far as the Key Area Handbook is concerned are

- Primary and secondary care
- NHS and local authority social service departments
- Voluntary sector organizations
- Education and youth services
- The housing sector
- The criminal justice system
- Employers and trades unions
- Employment services
- Local media

A range of possible interventions by these agencies and organizations is proposed to meet the strategic direction of the Health of the Nation and the mental illness targets (DOH 1993a) on suicide and social functioning. Examples of potential mental health-promoting activity will be developed under these headings in subsequent chapters.

Working Together for Better Health (DOH 1993c)

In the government document *Working Together for Better Health* the role of healthy alliances is given further emphasis. It is clear what the outcome of working together across professional and public boundaries can achieve. This is made evident in the foreword by the Secretary of State for Health: 'One of the key themes in *The Health of the Nation* is that by working together – in "healthy alliances" – we can all achieve more than we can by working separately. Working together we can better make sure that services and facilities are in place and used, that the environment in which we live, work and play is safe and conducive to health, and that people have the clear and consistent information they need to help themselves maintain and improve their health' (p.2). This sets the stall out for the remainder of the document, with an individualized focus on health prioritized. The main advances in health are said to be achievable by the following:

- Encouraging people themselves to lead healthier and safer lives and promoting the availability of affordable healthy choices: ***changing behaviour***
- Ensuring healthier and safer environments in which people can live, work and play: ***changing environments***
- Providing the right type of high-quality local services: ***providing better services***

Thus, we have behaviour and environment change and improved service provision as the platform on which to achieve a healthy population. At its most useful, the document gives advice on setting up healthy alliances, including challenges and ways to overcome them.

Fit for the Future (DOH 1995d)

This is the second progress report on the Health of the Nation. In its overview the report applauds the success of the national health strategy especially in terms of its widening: 'Health is no longer seen as the exclusive property of health professionals, hospitals, the NHS and the Department of Health' (p.7). It describes work in hand to develop work in 'healthy settings'. These include schools, hospitals, prisons, cities, homes, workplaces and environments. In terms of communicating the

Health of the Nation to the general population the following point is worth quoting; 'Effective communication of health messages is about *giving people information they need to make their own health choices*' (p.11, italics in original). The progress report also makes reference to the 'Health of the Young Nation' which is aimed at improving the health of young people and making sure they can make 'responsible choices about their health and lifestyle' (p.13).

The Health of the Nation – Key Area Handbook: Mental Illness (DOH 1993a) and associated documentation calls for a commitment to prevention and to the voluntary sector, but the emphasis remains on people with a mental illness, including prevention strategies targeted at the mentally ill rather than the general population. Here the emphasis is more about demystifying mental illness. How this can be squared with the emphasis placed on community treatment and a focus on the Mental Health Act remains difficult to see. From a public education perspective, attempting to destigmatize severe mental illness is a difficult if not impossible undertaking. As ever, what may be required is a more honest and fundamental discussion about the nature of mental illness, causation, contradictions in treatment interventions, including risks and alternatives, and a practical demonstration of what is expected of the public within a care framework evolving from normalization principles.

What then would such educational material consist of? We can look at the literature which critically explores the underlying ideologies of health education material and develop information that is explicit about the Mental Health Act, about normalization and about some of the dilemmas and contradictions surrounding treatment, rehabilitation and social support. There may also be room to discuss some of the negative aspects of mental illness as well as lessons learned in terms of the contribution that people with a long-term mental health problem can make to their own community, including responses via consultation processes to the services that are provided to help not just them but also, potentially, the whole community as and when required.

Public consultation

Rigge (1995) looks critically at public consultation in the NHS. She refers to the recent policy statement from the NHS Executive (1995), *Priorities and Planning Guidance for the NHS 1996–97*, Leeds. This emphasizes user involvement and patient empowerment. Good consumer involvement is complex and it costs. It is not something that can be undertaken lightly or with a minimal budget. As Rigge states, 'It requires strong commitment from board level down, and an organizational culture which regards proper consultation with users and would-be users as a vital part of quality service, not an optional occasional exercise.' She goes on to argue that consumers as well as staff need training and support and recommends the use of focus groups. This should be done in collaboration with community groups and advocacy services, if they exist. Self-help and voluntary organizations are also ways of accessing the public. Timing is also an issue in terms of need, giving the impression that the agenda, including the consultation process, is already set. This requires both forward thinking and planning and a need to be flexible enough to meet any views and changes which early discussion can have on the implementation of a consultation exercise. Confidentiality and anonymity as well as the location of the consultation process also need to be taken into account. And finally, feedback and involvement in shaping and informing the dissemination process after the consultation period as well as evaluation of the exercise itself are required. While this may seem overkill, this sort of investment will pay positive returns in future consultation exercises. The proper regard for and establishment of respect for and dialogue with a range of voluntary and user groups will be of benefit to the public and the professional services.

Conclusion

A health alliance approach to promoting mental health involves a recognition by the practitioner, whether as part of the statutory or mainstream health and social services, of the need to consider the views and experiences of the general public and service users. This process should also involve a host of other services and organizations to enhance and inform all service delivery on people's mental well-being. True consultation and community participation are key elements of a health alliance approach and ones which the practitioner can be positively engaged with.

According to government strategy, specialist mental health services should seek local views. The Health of the Nation – Key Area Handbook: Mental Illness (DOH 1993a) gives a checklist of what effective consultation means and what practical support is required in order to achieve this. Information is a dominant theme and practitioners are in a good position to work with people to develop a range of resources to inform the public and enable it to advocate for positive change on mental health issues. Despite the state's emphasis on consultation, there are areas of contention. The issue of management legitimizing and creating the right conditions for health and social care providers to engage in community participation processes is key. This is where organizational development work on the part of the statutory agencies is so vital in order to facilitate a climate in which staff as individuals and teams can fully pursue participation and the principles that underlie it.

Participation, in all its guises, is a pragmatic element of a health alliance approach and is a route to promoting mental health. It allows potential, existing and past users of all mental health services to inform and change practice. It enables the practitioner to consider other factors which influence mental illness, mental health and emotional well-being. It puts their practice and other agencies' practice in context and in perspective. Ultimately, if done correctly it should make professionals a little more modest and a lot more concerned about the views and ideas of their fellow citizens.

Practice checklist

- Familiarize yourself with the literature and documents that refer to community participation and health alliances to identify your role in the process.

- Identify existing local networks, forums and joint activity on mental health issues — are their any gaps, or key agencies or communities missing?

- Remember you are a citizen — how might you want to be consulted on a health issue?

Imagine yourself as newly arrived in a culture quite different from your own. You have mental health problems and limited funds and cannot speak the local language. What would you want from a health alliance? How would you want to be involved and helped to become involved in participation?

Identify a key agency and try and map out your own agency's actual and potential links with other services such as local media, welfare rights, day centres, and places of worship.

Think of ways in which you can nurture and sustain contacts with voluntary and user-led groups in the mental health field.

Strategy and strategic approaches

4

To borrow from Quinn (1992) an MHP strategy is . . . *the pattern or plan that integrates an organization's major goals, policies, and action sequences into a cohesive whole. A well formulated strategy helps to marshal and allocate an organization's resources into a unique and viable posture based on its relative internal competencies and shortcomings, anticipated changes in the environment, and contingent moves by intelligent opponents.* (Quinn 1992, in *The Strategy Process*)

Strategy is a popular word in modern management language. Although often presented as a complex concept, it can be simply described as a logical method for influencing and controlling the future but one which contains within itself the seeds of illogicality, since by the nature of the process a substantial amount of 'guessology' is brought into play. (Eskin 1992)

Key themes:

- Defining strategy and a strategic approach
- Strategy and MHP – how to influence it
- Examples of good practice

Overview

This chapter examines strategic approaches to mental health and its promotion. There is an acknowledgement that a strategic approach for mental health as well as for mental illness contains an element of systematic planning and lateral thinking, especially for people involved in service provision. The daily activity and relatively immediate responses and reactions required by professional and other staff to crises and calls for help may not appear to sit comfortably with this way of thinking. However, in order to support environments (and services) conducive to mental health as well as mental illness, cohesion and purposeful targeting are prerequisites. As in the other chapters, this will be done considering elements that make up a mental health-promoting framework in relation to

- The general public
- Voluntary agencies
- Professionals
- The state
- Health services
- Social services

Mental health promotion at the strategic level

What is a strategy?

A dictionary definition of strategy is that it is a plan of action or policy in business or in politics (*Oxford Modern English Dictionary*, 1993). The marketplace economics of health and social care, with mental health as a politically charged issue, make such a definition, however unintentionally, highly applicable to MHP. The purpose of a strategy can be said to be a process by which a group or organization sets out a possible plan for the future. Such a plan has as its framework:

1. A set of principles
2. A rationale for change
3. A set of objectives
4. Time scales to meet that change and
5. It acts as a blueprint for specific actions by services or agencies that can singularly or collectively achieve change.

A strategy may be broad, such as a National Health strategy, or more local, committing health and local authorities to joint action on, for example, the needs of carers. A strategic approach may be one that evolves from national policy and is spearheaded by statutory bodies or it may be in response to policy at local campaigning level. Thus, strategy is as much about the purpose and intention of action as it is a plan in itself. It may consist of an overall approach within a community development framework to lobby and campaign, for example on health issues such as water metering, poverty or access to transport. A key element of a strategy is the development of contacts, making allies and gaining cross-agency commitment on a range of activity. What a strategy consists of will vary but there will be common elements within a strategic plan whether it is nationally or locally based. Within a mental health perspective we have identified themes that can be considered for inclusion (Box 4.1). The list is not exhaustive and community participation as a process (see Chapter 3) should underpin it.

Box 4.1 **Themes to be included in a strategy**

- **A rationale:** Background information giving the reasons for producing a mental health strategy
- **An analysis of needs:** This may be statistical quantitative data and qualitative expressed needs of individuals, groups and communities
- **A stock take:** The context in which current services, support and activity in the mental health field take place. This can include what is available, its quality and relevance

- **Philosophy and principles:** The values and principles upon which the strategy is based
- **Aims:** What it is that those producing the strategy are trying to do
- **Actions, activities and methods:** How the aims can be achieved
- **Measurements and targets:** This will include monitoring and evaluation on achieving aims
- **Dissemination and implementation:** Gaining agreement, founding ownership and responding to views and comments of individuals, groups and organizations. An implementation process for a strategy may also include a costed operational plan for funding or reallocating funding to achieve the strategy's aims

Strategy and MHP

MHP has tended to operate within a broad canvas of projects and initiatives involving strategic planning of mental health services and community-based interagency work. This strategic level can include healthy city and healthy institution approaches to promoting overall population health and health strategies that are part of the responses to health and social policy more specifically within health and mental health. It is in the area of MHP at a strategic level that there is a possible synthesis of issues for the public, the professional mental health practitioners and the power of the state as mediated via professionals. Indeed, it is a strategic approach for the planning and activity, matched with a vision for the future direction of the mental health of the total population, that is required. This also includes the international level. Fernando (1993) suggests that the World Health Organization (WHO) needs to make a strategic shift in its approach to mental health: that is, to move away from projects that are aimed at the treatment of mental illness to ones which alleviate stress, especially in culturally specific domains. He also argues that WHO should focus on the development of 'indigenous methods of mental health promotion' utilizing local expertise in partnership with Western skills. As Westernized medical problem solving can be exported and imposed on other cultures, so too can mental health promotion strategies which fail to take account of the local conceptualization of and responses to mental health. As well as an explicit reference to the dangers of psychiatric or health-promoting 'colonialism', it also implies a need to consider community development approaches to health. This also leads us into the core aspect of any MHP strategy: that its context is social and therefore a social model of health is an inevitable and desirable consequence.

The other chapters map out the potential implementation, detail, dilemmas and pragmatic approaches to some of the concepts and ideas developed strategically. However, this should not presuppose that health and social care strategies produced at the local levels from broader national policy frameworks are simply imposed upon professionals and the public they serve. If this is the case the mental health services are no more than conduits for health and social policy. Their role is more crucial in taking forward strategy. It is in this middle ground in which the operational implementation of strategy can be sabotaged or can succeed. There are opportunities for the public, service users and carers and professionals to inform and influence strategy development and operational implementation of plans which can have positive and negative effects on the mental health of citizens. Whether this is in the shape of the large-scale shifts that Fernando refers to or at a more local scale of action is a double-edged sword. From the perspective of professionals it is in some senses also positive self-protection, as they are the group that will have to organize and deliver the themes and action of various strategies.

How can strategy be influenced?

We must accept that there are elements of strategy development and implementation requiring a pragmatic yet creative approach. In the field of existing strategies or health policy such as Health of the Nation and Community Care, interpretation is all. For example, care programming may be a convenient way of exerting degrees of control and ensuring compliance with packages of treatment and care. More positively, it allows opportunities for user and carer involvement in decision making. Therefore, even the most doctrinaire or apparently rigid strategy allows for opportunities for developing new ways of working and reflecting on the manner in which mental health practitioners plan and perform their tasks. This is difficult in a culture of change and resource constraint, but nevertheless is an opportunity for fundamental changes in attitudes and practices. There is also the issue of justification of MHP activity to one's managers: how to field and how to fashion action within your own work objectives. One way in which the practitioner can link into MHP at the strategic level is via policy and strategy developed by user and voluntary agencies, which are freer than the professional agencies to pursue a more holistic and socially based form of mental health. While practitioners in primary care, in social work or as part of a community mental health team may not be able to immerse themselves completely in what is described below, there are lessons to be learned and ideas to be shared. One example of users and the voluntary sector combining to develop a strategy for MHP is the framework developed by the North Western Mental Health Promotion Group (1994). This is an alliance of individuals and organizations committed to promoting mental health in the five metropolitan districts and four counties of northern England.

MHP – a framework (MINDS Matter)

The framework formulated by MINDS Matter has as its focus the general public and users of mental health services. A rationale for the framework is to maintain what it describes as 'a profile comparable to other health priorities in order that appropriate resources can be directed towards it'. The underlying philosophy of this strategy emanates from the Health for All movement, encompassing equity, participation and collaboration. At a practical level this is interpreted as:

- **Equity** – responses to inequalities in service provision and service access
- **Participation** – informing the public and involving them in planning
- **Collaboration** – interagency and professional and public cooperation

This framework sees mental health very much as a social product, stating positively that MHP should focus upon strengths rather than weaknesses of individuals and communities. Key to this is the concept of empowerment. Three areas are identified within the framework document:

- **Health education:** related to increasing people's skills in managing life events
- **Prevention:** assisting people in obtaining sufficient help and resources to support them through difficult times such as significant life events
- **Protection:** providing environments conducive to positive mental health

The work by Wycherley (1987) and Tannahill (1985) is drawn together to formulate these three areas of education, prevention and protection (see Chapter 6). In terms of the objectives that MINDS Matter has produced, these are translated into:

- **Education:** awareness of stress and responses to it, life skill training, assertiveness and coping strategies. An emphasis is placed on the school as a setting
- **Prevention:** self-help, development of self-esteem/acceptance
- **Protection:** housing, leisure and educational facilities. Encouraging employers to develop mental health policy, challenging stereotypes

These guidelines identify a process developing a MHP strategy, including supporting community development. This includes an ***assessment of need*** for the whole community utilizing quantitative and qualitative approaches. MINDs Matter identifies eight areas deemed important to include in a MHP strategy:

1. Raising public awareness of mental health
2. Promoting greater understanding of mental illness
3. Provision of comprehensive information to the public on the availability of mental health services, thereby enabling informed choice
4. Raising public awareness of how they might influence service delivery
5. Supporting the development of examples of good practice in the area of prevention
6. Involving and educating primary health care teams which have a key role to play in the field of mental health
7. Developing a resource base within a local area in the field of mental health promotion
8. Raising awareness among staff and elsewhere on both mental and physical health services of the principles of mental health promotion through the provision of conferences and workshops on specific topics.

All the issues above are ones that the mental health practitioner, either as part of mainstream services or otherwise, needs to be aware of. Many of the elements are within the scope, function, interest and requirements of a range of services including welfare rights agencies, supported accommodation projects, day care, primary care and specialist mental health teams. It is also important that workers who are part of community services, including practice and district nurses, health visitors, counsellors and associated primary care support agencies, also see themselves playing a role in the promotion of mental health as much as in the detection, treatment and care of ill-health.

The end result – outcomes

A measure of success for a strategy is whether the planning, 'guessology' and the implementation of how we see the future materialize in the way envisaged. The strategic outcomes of a given strategy will also tend to have a longer time scale than those of an annual business plan or annual planning and financial cycle. Despite this time scale there remain opportunities within a strategic framework to consider the outcomes of what a collection of activity will result in. This is important to secure credibility, funding and further resources, and to reflect and celebrate a sense of achievement on reaching milestones and overall change. The research by Macdonald (1994) is a national project commissioned by the Health Education Authority to identify evaluation methods used in MHP. While the area examined was primarily that of health promotion specialists and units developing and delivering a range of activity, there are significant implications for other professional staff within a strategy context.

The intention of the research was threefold: (1) reflection on the reasons why evaluation in this area is problematic; (2) an examination of the issues involved; and (3) identification of the practitioner's needs in the evaluation process. MacDonald demonstrated that while project development was an important part of mental health promotion, resulting from a 'community' needs assessment process, such assessment tended to be informal and undetermined. Many initiatives were based on assumptions about interventions to promote mental health without systematic assessment of need. The reasons for this were viewed as pragmatic as much as philosophical. There was a recognition that a formal needs assessment process can result in reactive and narrow service provision and in itself can raise false expectations. This has implications for a strategic approach to MHP, as assessment of need has been seen as a vital element. However, such assessment can be user- and community-focused, as demonstrated in Chapter 3. MacDonald also refers to the 'balloons or strategy' dilemma which MHP workers and, we would argue, all MHP can find itself in: that is, reactive health education-focused activity as against longer term interagency development and planning.

This is echoed in the recent review of MHP work by Monach and Spriggs (1995), who raise the following question:

> The elaboration of the purchaser/provider split required by recent health and community care legislation was seen as a tension for MHP, as it is for health promotion as a whole. Is it a service being provided as part of overall health provision, or is it a contribution to the decision making processes whereby strategic decisions are made as to which services should be purchased or what requirements should be built into contracts? (pp. 55–6).

They conclude with the telling remark that as the purchasing scenario develops, the complex role of MHP workers operating for trusts and health commissions may make such roles problematic. This is equally applicable to all health and social care professionals engaged in mental health-promoting initiatives. A strategic response to mental health requires a high degree of interagency exchange and collaboration. This does not sit easily with the market economy model which exists within health and social care currently predominating in the United Kingdom. Territorialism, competition and frequent organizational and role change are added challenges to a long-term approach to promoting mental health. However, strategic alliances have overcome such

How could you become involved in the development of strategy and how could you encourage others to do likewise?

Can the would-be mental health promoter influence the strategic direction of mental health policy and practice professionally (from within) or as part of a health alliance or ally of the public and the service user?

difficulties, as demonstrated with the Healthy City movement across the United Kingdom, Europe and beyond.

We now turn our attention to an examination of current national health strategy by looking at issues of inequality and health contained in *Variations in Health* (DOH 1995c)

Public health programmes and health strategy: *Variations in Health*

This document (DOH 1995c) provides guidance on interventions within the NHS to address variations in health status. It was developed using a survey of NHS Public Health Departments. The responses indicate eight elements of public health advocacy that could impact on health inequalities:

- Health needs assessment
- Local target setting
- Access to effective health care provision
- Alliances
- Resource allocation
- Purchasing by primary health care services
- Public health programmes
- The NHS as employer

Many of these elements would relieve the concerns expressed by MacDonald in that they provide a broad set of actions, which, in a strategic combination, can clarify MHP interventions. For our purposes the area of public health requires further scrutiny as it is another essential ingredient of a strategic approach to mental health promotion. Also, responses to strategies that the mental health promoter may encounter, become part of, or initiate are often public health initiatives. Whether this response takes the form of a public discussion, reproduction and dissemination of information, or is focused on population prevention strategies, it is important to highlight it given the significance that is placed on such approaches by government agencies and professionals themselves. Apart from perceived wisdom, there is little in the form of formulated education theory and evidence to support individual interventions. This assumes such activity to be a good thing in itself and, as it is time limited, to be worthy of some limited staff time input. A lack of a strategic vision at policy, management and operational levels excludes a combination of methods formulated as part of a consistent plan in order to achieve positive change. As part of a public health programme, *Variations in Health* gives examples of possible interventions together with positive and negative features of a public health programme. This is of great value in considering such an approach in the field of mental health promotion. The following are included as examples of interventions:

- Community participation
- Health information
- Community transport
- Welfare benefit provision within health settings
- Social support
- Use of the media
- Service specifications for interagency work by health promotion units
- Targeting of health promotion in settings
- Multiple setting community-based health promotion

It is acknowledged that the health service has over twenty years of experience of trying out small-scale projects with combinations of the above. What is now required, it states, is 'a policy commitment to adopting these methods through allocation of mainstream resources, and planned changes to professional practice and training of NHS staff to work effectively with more disadvantaged groups' (p.46). This is as important to the non-state and non-NHS sector as it is to that potential resource for promoting mental health – the infrastructure, skills and staff of the NHS.

The following are suggested features that mental health promoters need to consider in their work around a public health programme:

- Building self-confidence and self-esteem through experiential learning
- Understanding people's beliefs, the context and opportunities for change
- Offering practical support which is realistic and feasible
- Helping people to define for themselves what changes they would like to make and enabling them to gain access to information and advice about how to make those changes
- Promoting a positive and holistic view of health
- Providing opportunities for social integration through events, groups, informal contacts
- Acting as advocates on behalf of particular communities when appropriate
- Facilitating access to a variety of services and benefits

This is a possible checklist for informing a strategic framework that can address the mental health needs of the general population, of vulnerable elements of that population, and of the mentally ill themselves and doing so within a social framework. It also has consequences for strategic educational programmes which may be proposed within the mental illness and mental health fields.

The document goes on to give a salutary list of methods which are *ineffective* in enabling individuals and communities to strengthen social support. Many are familiar, especially to the communities and their supporters who have often had to suffer overzealous attempts at influencing health in the short term. Developers of mental health promotion strategies can learn a lot from reflection on such a list. *Ineffective* methods and ones to be wary of and to avoid include:

- Victim-blaming approaches
- Reinforcement of fatalism and a sense of despair
- Raising expectations that something might happen when the authorities have no intention of doing anything; surveys of disadvantaged people may be unethical and breed profound cynicism
- Leaving behind no locally sustainable infrastructure, resources or capability for community action in the longer term
- Offering a one-dimensional response to multiple health needs
- Offering a one-dimensional response to multiple health needs leading to isolation or exclusion

These ineffective methods are important to consider if public health approaches to, for example, a public education strategy for the detection, treatment and management of depression are to be successfully implemented (see Chapter 6).

A whole range of programmes, projects or initiatives woven together and based on a systematic assessment of community needs could be said to constitute a strategy for promoting mental health. In order to qualify for this, other factors need to be taken into consideration. From a strategic perspective we also ask 'Do we accept biomedical categories of mental illness and add social understandings to them, or proceed from a different premise?' The danger remains that approaches can be simple refinements and adjustments of the standard psychiatric paradigm. A strategic approach to mental health as well as mental illness should address this dilemma. As part of a community-focused, broad agency involvement, the very process of strategic mental health ensures that it is not the prevailing mental illness approaches that are prioritized. By thinking strategically we can and must include a range of actions, agencies and approaches that go beyond the narrow confines of specialist mental health provision.

Psychiatry recognizes that mental health problems arise from a complex background in which biological, psychological and social factors interact. The result has been an ever-expanding range of services, now most often located in non-hospital settings. There is also a shift towards more active user involvement and participation in care and rehabilitation. This is mirrored in government policy emphasizing the importance of health alliances and alternative management and intervention strategies to enable and 'empower' users and carers of psychiatric services. All this is to be welcomed, but there is a danger as part of this 'consumerism' of mental health that it becomes an individual possession to be improved by a range of services. This fits neatly into the revealing ideological orthodoxy expressed within the national health strategy and we need to be careful in order not to fall into the trap of simply providing more and more specialist services for problems which are social problems and the treatment of which requires social action. Mental illness is not inherent in individuals, rather it is produced by social and economic circumstances, increasing the risks of ill-health for some groups.

An example of a mental health strategy attempting to address both mental illness and mental health prevention and promotion can be found at the national level in The Health of the Nation.

The state: *Key Area Handbook: Mental Illness*

The Health of the Nation – *Key Area Handbook: Mental Illness* (DOH 1993a) suggests five broad themes which can be said to be strategic objectives for mental health promotion at the individual, group and agency level.

1. Reducing the incidence of mental illness and suicide by the ability to cope in stressful situations
2. Countering fear, ignorance and stigma about mental illness and creating a more positive social climate in which it becomes more acceptable to talk about feelings, emotions and problems. It is also to seek help without fear of labelling or feeling a failure.
3. Preventing the deterioration of an existing mental illness.
4. Improving the quality of life of people with long-standing, recurrent or acute mental health problems. This includes their families and friends.
5. Maintaining and improving social functioning

Achieving these five goals is very much within the sphere of a proactive approach to the issue of users, carers and their friends or allies. Despite these worthy statements, this strategy concentrates more on the vulnerable, the socially isolated, or those experiencing ill-health at an individual level than it does in trying to address structural factors which can hinder positive mental health for the population. In terms of the level identified by Whitehead as described in Chapter 1, it is at levels 1 and 2.

The key area also states that unlike treatment measures which can be immediate in their effect, health promotion is a longer-term strategy (p.27). From this perspective the following interventions and their effects are proposed:

1. Increasing awareness about mental illness
2. Changing public attitudes
3. Improving coping abilities in stressful situations
4. Countering the fear, ignorance and stigma which surround mental illness.

Thus, what is required is a 'longer-term strategy'. While there are fairly immediate measures that can be taken, such as information and service quality changes, the focus is on the medium to long term. The development of a MHP strategy in this document is to increase awareness of mental illness, changing public attitudes and developing preventive approaches (strategies). Again this is undetermined. Where do we start? Do we start with preventive, possibly small-scale measures in the form of projects and remoulding of existing service provision? One of the answers could lie in the political and reforming changes that have taken place within the health and social services sector. The other is the economic reality of forming and sustaining interprofessional activity, which in many senses parallels the time scale which health promotion, as a longer-term strategy, expects to deliver. In the short to medium term the professional groups are expected to initiate active networking with a range of key personnel and organizations to be drawn upon and to be mutually available. The reality is that this requires at the very minimum a degree of time commitment if it is to be planned, if it is to be effective and if it is to be valued. You would need to consider your role, understanding and commitment to strategic development.

Guidelines for strategy

Taking account of the above examples and discussion, it is possible to synthesize various elements into a framework to aid awareness of strategy content, its structure and possible intervention points for influence. *Guidelines for the Mental Health Promoter: A Strategic Approach to MHP* (G. McCulloch and J. Boxer, unpublished data) requires the practical points set out in Table 4.1. In short, a strategic approach to MHP is evolutionary and requires a synthesis of these three elements: the public, the professional and the state.

Table 4.1
Theory and practice framework for a strategic approach to MHP

Theory	Practice
An understanding of contemporary health and social strategy at national and local levels	Reviewing and clarifying existing policy and programmes that may have a mental health element
A readiness to examine and set outcome indicators	Looking at medium-term and long-term goals
An awareness and preparedness to use theory and models that have proved effective in other settings	Becoming aware of health promotion theory and practice, tapping into existing units and university and research settings
Interagency dialogue and cooperation linking into existing structures	Identifying existing consultation processes, health and community forums, and sharing common areas of concern and possible mutual problem solving for organizations – e.g. linking into church organizations around mental health issues
Addressing the local agenda within your own discipline or interest area; sounding out colleagues and other groups	Making use of what good relationships between agencies you have and nurturing them. What are the existing discussion groups and forums where mental health can be an agenda item?
Utilizing existing quantitative and qualitative data and material on health and mental health	Checking out a range of research from health, housing, social services and universities. Highlighting gaps in research on areas you find important
Establishing and maintaining contacts with as wide a range of the general public as possible	This includes users, carers, voluntary agencies and organizations such as Community Health Councils, tenants' associations and various working parties
'Costing' and negotiating agreement on which agencies will take the lead in what areas.	What are agencies prepared to offer in terms of changing culture and practice and reconfiguring and reorienting services to take account of mental health issues, e.g. Mental Health at Work policy development or specialist mental health nurse liaison with primary care teams?

Cross-strategy awareness

There are a range of strategic plans and approaches which may impact directly or indirectly on people's mental and emotional well-being. As such they have the capacity to promote mental health, or they can be influenced to take into account mental health as well as, when appropriate, mental ill-health. These need to considered and worked through as part of formulating or working on existing strategy development. They also have consequences and effects. Transport and housing strategy, for example, can have considerable impact on mental health as well as other environmental factors.

It is also important to consider existing strategies which may relate directly or indirectly to mental health. There are opportunities to become involved in and shape other health and related strategies which may have a direct or indirect bearing on people's mental health (see Box 4.2).

Box 4.2 **A list of possible national and more local strategies**

- Healthy Cities strategies, City Challenge, Single Regeneration Budget and Urban Renewal strategies
- Home Office Tackling Drugs Together initiative
- Annual purchasing plans of health authorities and business plans of trusts and GP fundholders
- Community Care plans
- Joint finance and other funding criteria
- Sexual health strategies
- Children's Act/Children plan
- Housing policy
- Disability Act
- Local considerations such as rural or town settings, age and ethnic population

Conclusion

Mainstream psychiatry recognizes that mental health problems have a complex background in which biological, psychological and social factors interact. A strategic approach is, therefore, a necessity when considering mental illness and mental health. However, the state's responses to this can be an increasing array of professionals, models and theories attempting to treat the mentally ill fairly or democratically. This has even reached the point at which government policy strives to argue for the importance of health alliances and alternative management and interventions to enable and empower users and carers in the psychiatric arena. Mental health can become, like everything else, an individual possession to be improved by a range of services. This fits comfortably into prevailing ideologies embedded within the national health strategy. The mental health promoter, as specialist or generalist in the mental health field needs to be aware of this. Failure to do so may result in the provision of more specialist services for what are social problems requiring social action to be resolved. A strategic approach offers opportunities and also raises concerns. Many of the examples discussed remain focused on mental illness rather than on mental health. Involvement in the process of strategy, at whatever levels, must ensure that this agenda is given the prominence it deserves. Genuine long-term changes, shifts in public attitude and good community health require plans, schemes and input from a host of agencies and organizations. There are many avenues open for dialogue, interagency work and innovative partnerships. However, networking, liaison and the fostering of good relationships with a host of other organizations are seldom taken into account when it comes to quantifying the input of workers. Such involvement also can take people away from their core activity. It is for this reason that levels of involvement in any mental health promotion strategy, actual or potential, should be made clear. Further, the core tasks of all the stakeholders in mental health should be defined and refined to include their contribution to the process.

Practice checklist

- Identify the points of entry for service users. Is it their advocate or the professional supporter who influences and informs strategy?

- Are users only involved when it comes to consultation? Identify mechanisms in which users of your service can become involved.

- Is the professional equally marginalized from the development of strategy? Look at current strategies: see the overlaps, gaps and areas that are relevant to your practice.

- What would you suggest to enable more practitioner and service recipient involvement in strategic planning and purchasing/commissioning?

- Would focus groups be one way of using existing client case work and opportunistic discussion? How would you 'record' this in order to capture views, ideas and testimony? Are there ethical considerations in the capture and use of such material?

- What happens if the service user viewpoint runs counter to that of the professionals and their employees and policy makers? It is important to develop contacts with the voluntary and user sectors to have these debates in the open.

- What are the ethical implications of designing and implementing a mental health promotion strategy?

Education and training

5

*With progressive education, respect for the knowledge of living experience
is inserted into the larger horizon against which it is generated – The
horizon of cultural context, which cannot be understood apart from its
class particularities, and this indeed in societies so complex that the
characteristics of those particularities is less easy to come by.*
(Friere 1996, p.85)

Key themes:

- Rationale (Chapters 1 and 9)
- Political and educational context (Chapters 1, 2, 6 and 9)
- Where is the theory? (Chapters 1 and 9)
- Practice within statutory provision (Chapter 7)
- Practice in the voluntary and private domains: relationships with
  professionals (Chapters 3 and 8)
- User involvement and advocacy (Chapters 8 and 10)
- Community as a setting, a resource and underpinning social
  participation (Chapter 3)

Overview

This chapter considers the parameters for education and training in
mental health promotion and in informing eclectic and interdisciplinary
curriculum development and innovative practice. It is therefore the key

chapter for students and mental health practitioners to consider their role and function in relation to the key themes.

Rationale

It is probably unrealistic to think that one model or framework for education and training could encompass all the knowledge and experience required for engaging in the process of increasing emotional and social well-being or promoting mental health in the context we have identified. Mental health promotion has mainly developed as a core aspect within the framework of health promotion and education but it is redefining its boundaries all the time. It has also been an identified component of the teaching of mental health practice for many years, although not as explicitly defined as it is now.

The state now has a more vested interest in health as a commodity and, to a limited extent, in the way policies inform an educational and training agenda. At the same time as we would wish to put mental health promotion more firmly on the map, some parallel understanding is necessary in determining:

- The extent to which the historical context of the treatment of mental illness still has a negative effect on current practice and cannot be avoided
- The extent to which the socio-cultural-economic position of large groups of people as disadvantaged, oppressed and alienated all too often still determines any diagnosis of mental illness

Mental health promotion has to be realized primarily in the 'public' arena, and this aspect, while not negating the role of professionals, is the greatest challenge. The evidence is that past health education and promotion strategies, in terms of public perception of what does us harm, have not been very popular or successful, and have certainly not brought about a strong enough rationale for change. The 'way' things are taught in this domain, professionals being part of this public we identify, is crucial and probably more important than the content. Our experience of teaching mental health promotion over the last six years has been to 'liberate' mental health from being just the other end of the spectrum from mental illness, or an ideal state, and to position ourselves and our experience with others in a more equitable and manageable way. Psychiatry, in its attempts to straddle both medical and social models of practice, has to a large extent ignored the latter approach. The role and function of this discipline has its basis in the moral, legal and statutory authority of itself as the main professional group caring for the mentally ill. It would seem to have very little time for the practical necessity of promoting mental health, choosing rather to want confirmation of cause and diagnosis. Nor is mental health a permanent state which can be 'treated', however much identified problems are considered in terms of traditional notions of 'ill-health'. It would seem that we cannot escape dichotomous relationships and power imbalances, however much we want to increase our knowledge about this subject. There are exceptions, and any reading of radical, anti- and transcultural psychiatry exposes major flaws and considers fundamental dilemmas about the nature and practice of traditional psychiatry (Fernando 1991).

If we are seeing a real change towards collaborative interagency and interdisciplinary practice, it has been a long time coming and still has a long way to go (Hornby 1993). Abundant statistics, media portrayal and accounts of personal tragedy highlight the acute link between ill-health, mental illness and levels of unemployment, poverty and deprivation as being so interwoven that they can no longer be dismissed as useful ammunition for left-wing 'hype'. Obviously one cannot ignore the necessity of a statutory framework for mental illness and the limited need for secure provision, ECT, and seclusion. What is perhaps needed is a more explicit approach which would include, at all stages of education and training, the need to assess mental health in a positive framework which does not ignore the multiplicity of factors which have contributed to an unstable perspective of the world and how one relates to others in it (Dalley 1996).

We accept that mental health promotion is a nebulous concept that can change in perspective as soon as one thinks one has grasped its meaning and value. There will always be the problem of assessing its relevance to the more powerful concept of mental illness and to the psychiatric system. Mental illness has an identity, it can be categorized and made part of the structure of any given society or institutional system, thereby somehow justifying its existence. There is no such justification for mental health. No one really knows what this desired goal is, or why it is so important, however many philosophers and theorists have dissected its meaning and value and tried to synthesize its essence as a meaningful 'whole'. We know that culturally there are enormous differences in the way mental health and illness are understood and 'treated' and how hard it is to incorporate this diversity into mainstream education. The overlaying of racism, sexism, poverty and class-based practices has led to enormous debates about 'which came first' in determining why so many people have more than one struggle in their life in trying to maintain positive mental health. The unconditional acceptance and inclusion of people from different ethnic or cultural backgrounds, who can inform educational initiatives as well as policy and practice, is an emerging element of current mental health practice and is to be welcomed and encouraged. This represents a positive outcome in terms of an educational strategy for mental health promotion.

We can probably only enhance our understanding and a value base to practice, which underpins any notion of social justice, by engaging in a more equitable process of acquiring knowledge and competence in this domain (Dominelli 1997a). Primarily, as stated, this resides in the 'public' arena, and in terms of critical education and education within primary health and social care (Green *et al.* 1996). In terms of mental health promotion, we can only develop our practice when we grow and engage with others in forms of relationships different from those we have now:

> It is not enough to keep practising the wrong done by others. More CPNs [community psychiatric nurses] could try to stop the damage in the first place, by being confident that what you have to offer is, above all, humanity and respect for fellow citizens. (Lindow 1996, p.8)

A very useful critique of these concerns is presented in a recent book that highlights the fundamental problem of incompatible values in social work (Banks 1995). The practice of social work, especially for an approved social worker, has always been caught in the dichotomy of being a movement towards social justice while at the same time having to act as a statutory agent of social control and community regulation. This account mirrors the same problematic in mental health nursing, especially in any consideration of the relationship between values, knowledge and skill in the development of ethical practice. Some theoretical consideration needs to be given to the problematic of what constitutes 'competence', as this has major implications for how the 'public' realize any notion of 'autonomy'. The development not only of an ethics of justice but also of an ethics of care is needed to inform these debates, and we are acutely aware of the enormity of what is constituted by this framework (Tronto 1993).

The teaching of mental health promotion is therefore as diverse as it has to be specific to:

- Culturally, community and politically based educational approaches which see mental health as a litmus test of one's socioeconomic position in any given culture or society
- Small-scale interventions at the level of one-to-one relationships inextricably bound up in the domains of psychiatry and statutory mental health provision

Political and educational context: value base to practice

Before examining the relationship of education and training to specific roles and situated experience, it is important to have some knowledge of education and its philosophical roots, its meaning and value. Although mental health promotion is considered at the level of primary, secondary and tertiary approaches, perhaps it is within the domain of primary health and social care relationships that investment in education can have most impact. If there is one writer who is most referred to in radical and political approaches to education it is Paulo Friere. Friere's contribution, although based on experiences in Latin America, is transferable and is illuminating in placing education in its most relevant context.

> My ethical duty, as one of the agents, of a practice that can never be neutral – the educational – is to express my respect for differences in ideas and positions. I must respect even positions opposed to my own, positions that I combat earnestly and with passion . . . Hence the watchfulness with which progressive educators ought to act . . . Hence the exigency they must impose on themselves of growing ever more open and forthright, of turning ever more critical, of becoming ever more curious. (Friere 1996, p.80)

The following matrices highlight major theoretical and practice issues to consider. Discuss with colleagues and educators how mental health promotion could be realized in this adaptation as an educational premise and related to primary health care. Who are the experts in this and why?

Identified 'components' of a philosophy of primary health care with suggested examples of how premises might be drawn from writings of Paulo Friere (Macdonald and Warren 1991)

A BASIC NORMATIVE PREMISES	B BASIC FACTUAL PREMISES
Education should be an act of liberation for the person . in community	The situation of oppression is the fact of lifefor many people in the world today.
Education should *empower* people. people.	Human beings have the ability to overcome their oppression.

C DISPOSITIONS TO BE FOSTERED	D METHODOLOGICAL PREMISES
Natural curiosity is the major feature to be fostered in people together with an assertive critically enquiring outlook.	Real-learning is done in a context of active, cooperative self-directed interaction.

| An acceptance of learning as dialogue. | Real-learning involves a problem-posing methodology that is inseparable from action. |

E
RECOMMENDATIONS FOR PRACTICE

Learning must start from people's own knowledge and build on their strengths – more questioning than answering by a 'teacher' conceived as a facilitator rather than an imparter of knowledge.

The practice of education is to be one of dialogue between partners regarded as equals.

The 'components' and examples of premises of a philosophy of primary health care as might be drawn from the writings of Paulo Friere (Macdonald and Warren 1991)

A BASIC NORMATIVE PREMISES	B BASIC FACTUAL PREMISES
Primary health care should be viewed as an educative process whereby people acquire greater control over their own lives.	Most ill-health has its roots in socio-economic conditions often created by exploration and its consequences in the unjust distribution of health resources.
C DISPOSITIONS TO BE FOSTERED	D METHODOLOGICAL PREMISES
People will be adept at discovering the cause and solutions for ill-health rather than content with merely addressing symptoms.	Genuine education for health can be shown to be more than a mere transfer of information but rather to involve a genuine encouragement of people's confidence in their ability to improve their own health.

E
RECOMMENDATIONS FOR PRACTICE

Learning about health will start from people's own knowledge and experience of health and disease. The wider social and political context will be a primary rather than a peripheral consideration in a dialogic interaction between parties construed as 'equal' but 'different' in relation to health concerns as they arise.

Macdonald and Warren's critique of a model for education and primary health care is useful at many levels. It questions the fundamental nature and experience of education and health, and does have a 'truly educative dimension'; also it ' . . . shifts concerns from a narrower "primary medical care" emphasis, which too easily can be 'merely' a training exercise' (Macdonald and Warren 1991, p.48).

To utilize this level of sophistication in such analysis allows for, and can provide the practitioner with, a conceptual critical 'toolbox' to employ with other elements in their practice. In mental health nursing this has been obscured because of the powerful element of 'therapy' as the defining role, and the development of professional nursing practice steeped in the theories and models of general nursing, especially from an American perspective. For the profession of social work, the recent change in the Central Council for Education and Training in Social Work's (CCETSW) antiracist and language policies is seen as a retrograde step in terms of this national body really being ' . . . a racially sensitive and culturally aware organization' (Lynn and Muir 1996). This will be discussed further in the section which looks at the development of anti-oppressive practice, but consideration of these points is highly relevant in terms of what the public, professionals and the state want and our basic rights and responsibilities towards education and health concerns.

Such a vision obviously requires immense commitment and competence. Engagement with others in experiential learning in the political and social context of diverse perspectives on health and illness is not the main focus of most educational establishments. At the present there is much debate about where mental health and learning disability, as branches of nursing within a Project 2000 model, can be best placed to fulfil these requirements. At the time of writing this book, intense debate and counter-argument has being going on about the relevance of sociology to the practice of nursing (Morrall 1996). Social work has considered this as integral to identifying the problematics of welfare, and in identifying why we have such a problem with the theory/practice divide. This has been considered, according to Dominelli (1997a), since the early 1990s as part of the development of voluntary work by the Charity Organization Society.

> . . . sociological social work aims to identify and disentangle the politics of practice, thereby enabling us to take more rational decisions about social work activities from a humanistic position which is concerned with facilitating an individual's capacity to develop his or her full potential for growth

in a society which acknowledges interdependence as part of the covenant between the individual and the state. (Dominelli 1997a, p.2)

Unfortunately, these fundamental issues are being overshadowed by the massive economic cuts being experienced at all levels of education. The basics, such as the right environment, time, motivation, and sound academic and practice outcomes, are being obscured by the necessity for large numbers of students within limited provision. At the present time there are thousands of carers and health and social care assistants working in all areas of mental health practice who have limited access to education and training initiatives, yet these are the ones most likely to have to cope with very difficult and complex needs, often without the experience to do so. Our experience of the introduction of NVQ standards for competence is that they have limited scope and rely too much on a few trained verifiers to fulfil such diverse requirements. A major problematic, as identified by Lewis and Glennerster (1996) is the increasingly artificial divide between health and social care and the immense damage that poorly thought out policies are doing to welfare provision in the late 1990s.

> What few proponents do is face up to the fundamental illogicality of the present divide between NHS and local authority funding and all the petty boundary disputes to which this gives rise . . . . It is not merely more money, public and private, that the services need, but a saner way of bridging the divide between 'free'(centrally tax-funded) health care and means-tested and locally funded social care.' (Lewis and Glennerster 1996, p.20a)

These authors do not consider educational needs as the primary focus of their book and we would question where and how this is being addressed in current state policies and by awarding bodies such as the English National Board (ENB) and CCETSW and in further and higher education.

Where is the theory?

> The object ought not to be to 'know', but to schematize: to impose as much regularity and form upon chaos as our practical needs require. (Nietzsche, in Stoddard, 1993)

If we are to be more explicitly involved in education and training in relation to MHP, there has to be an identification and analysis of current debates about the theories which underpin it. Tudor's (1996) book on MHP and highly informative articles in journals such as *Health Promotion International* both highlight a dilemma and level of complexity which cannot be ignored (Kelleher 1996).

Since the late 1970s the development of health promotion has gained great momentum. Obviously it is not the panacea for determining the 'health of the nation', but it has had enormous impact in informing how individual and societal health is realized and enacted. At the level of education and training this is a highly complex and possibly contentious issue. There seems to be great difficulty in realizing a theoretical basis to mental health promotion which can somehow span the conceptual tensions between the sociological paradigms of Burrell and Morgan and the way it has been further conceptualized by Caplan and Holland (1990). This needs to be considered alongside the more traditional models or approaches to this subject. The main elements of these paradigms would seem to be as follows.

1. The *functionalist paradigm* comprises the dominant view in medicine and sociology of maintaining equilibrium as equating to health and the justification to regulate behaviour considered 'deviant'
2. The *interpretative paradigm* comprises thoughts and ideas which attempt to understand and explain the social world from subjective experience
3. The *radical humanist paradigm* is the emphasis on subjectivity and a critique of the process of change at macro and micro levels of societal arrangements and human interaction
4. The *radical structuralist paradigm* is concerned with offering alternatives and puts in context the key problematic of relationships at the individual and social levels of interaction

Practitioners can locate themselves within the various paradigms and axes to determine the dominant social theory at any given time, as a guide and to enhance knowledge. The concern is that these paradigms are fixed states which do not identify the dialectical tensions inherent within the remit of practitioners, on the one hand working with a structuralist paradigm involving the Mental Health Act and the science of psychiatry, but on the other as citizens as well as practitioners, lobbying and activating for social justice within the community in which they live and work. Macdonald (1994) in his research on mental health promotion practice highlighted a lack of theoretical robustness. He argues that the model proposed by Caplan and Holland was useful in developing, implementing and evaluating MHP programmes and initiatives, but questions the 'newness' and theoretical validity of these paradigms.

The strength of Caplan and Holland's work is that it is accessible in providing an opportunity for analysis of the wider structural factors which limit and influence these paradigms. It can be empowering for practitioners themselves to be enabled by a theoretical model which forms the basis of a more thorough examination of the causes and consequences of mental ill-health and its management. This in turn allows opportunities for identifying ways of promoting mental health and an identified element of action to this process. As Banks, in her recent book on ethics and values, points out: ' . . . For Friere, reflection without action results in "mentalism", and action without reflection in "activism"; and both are empty' (Banks 1995, p.49). It also frees the practitioner to acknowledge the extent and possibility of involvement at micro and macro levels and to realize one's individual or group position in this. For communities and communities of interest it can allow a clearer exploration of the power and control inherent in mental health practice.

This, in our minds, has to be supported with current informative and relevant activities by 'nonprofessionals', such as people working in user service-led initiatives at the level of statutory as well as voluntary provision (Barnes and Wistow 1990; Beresford 1990). This begs the question of the extent to which defined or professional roles within the domain of health and social care can any longer be the main determining feature. In our account, MHP is clearly defined as the *action* element of any representational framework of our understanding of health and illness. This action should be based not on the need to delineate boundaries and continue professional rivalry but rather to enhance social participation and connectedness whatever the locality, and primarily as 'caring' human beings (Rudman 1996). This is a highly complex issue at both macro and micro levels of analysis and discourse in this field.

Another important, and neglected, aspect of theory development, especially in nursing education, is the way in which ideology maintains the illusion of power and oppression which so dominates modern society and sets people with similar wants and needs against each other (MIND 1995). We have mentioned critical education as being relevant to our discussions and would now add to this critical social theory as a core subject of study and debate in mental health promotion. Tudor provides an account of radical practice in his book which further explores the point we are making in terms of the theories which have informed that practice (Tudor 1996, p.211). More pragmatically, our social experience through desire for 'community' life cannot be adequately defined or critiqued, as much as we would like, in terms of abstract representation and the relevance of post-modern accounts. We realize that for the vast majority of the public it might be better to start with a more realistic and common understanding of health and illness, and of social policy/administration and its impact on community welfare, and argue that case first! (Tudor 1996; Humphries 1996). For those who wish to develop their ideas further, in Chapter 10 we have highlighted some accounts of ideology as points of discussion and debate. The following quotation indicates how important and central this subject is:

. . . ideology is the social cement of human society. It positions human subjects at a place where ideological meanings are constituted and thereby structures the real organization of social relations. It establishes, in sum, the deeply pervasive and unconscious modes by which subjects come to 'live out' their real relations to society. (Elliott 1992, p.165)

Dalrymple and Burke (1995), whose recent contribution in the area of anti-oppressive practice we discuss in the next section, highlight the work of Smid and Van Krieken in developing a typology of three levels of understanding in the complex relationship between theory and practice in health and social care. We support this identification and would encourage readers to consider this account:

Material social theory – gives an overview of how society is organized – consensus and conflict explanations of society.
Strategic practice theory – challenges the problematic of how to do things, especially if government rhetoric is to 'build bridges' and forge positive partnerships in care.
Working concepts – realizing the nature of power within the organizations where we are oppressed and consideration of how these affect and reflect on our practice. (Dalrymple and Burke 1995, p.10)

The pertinence of this typology for training, education and MHP is considerable and it raises numerous questions for the practitioner.

How important is theory in informing competent practice?

What responsibility do you think you have in effecting change in terms of mental health promotion?

In your chosen discipline, how do you think mental health promotion should be taught and by whom?

What aspect of community development and participation would you feel most 'powerful' in and why?

If you had to think of an action plan to implement a strategy for mental health promotion in your educational or practice setting, how would you go about this?

Practice within statutory provision

The practitioner looking for universal features or factors in the otherwise highly individual fabric or emotional distress is undoubtedly laying essential foundations for a more scientific approach to understanding psychopathology. But those who by virtue of particular theoretical commitments to the presumed 'disorder' never really see the client as a person with his or her own stories and theories are neither good therapists nor good scientists . . . .

This way we may come closer to offering our clients a 'good-enough' therapeutic space, within which to explore the meaning of their experiences. In
the end, all our observations of psychopathology can only inform us about a
part of a person and, even if accurate, they should never be divorced from
the socio-cultural context in which the person lives. (Lemma 1996, p. 23)

There is an 'assumed', rather than a covert, acceptance within the confines of the psychiatric paradigm that the factors determining mental
ill-health are the big social issues of unemployment, inequality and
oppressions of various kinds. There may even be a willingness to debate
and act upon the edges of these issues, such as by improving access to
welfare rights for people who use mental health services. However, the
'global' extent of the social and economic factors which impinge on
mental health can be seen as too broad, too abstract at a macro level to
respond to. Similarly to the arguments put forward against looking at
health from an international perspective, there is a reluctance to engage
in the roots and circumstances which inhibit health potential/gain:

If only people would engage in practices and behaviours which are health
promotive, the thinking went, there would be an immense decrease in
human suffering. Some were even more sanguine, promising an increase
in human happiness, as if health were the only aspect of human existence
determinant of happiness. (Antonovsky 1996,p.12)

Exposing the political and economic context allows services to become
aware of their ideological stake and options for change or influence.
The tension for the practitioner, although it remains, can be identified,
acknowledged and negotiated in terms of possible interventions and
actions within different paradigms. This is most obvious in the personal
and professional divide that practitioners experience. It is more than
simply wearing different 'hats' for different occasions. It spells out the
contradictions and opportunities in the mental health field and
identifies important choices to be made. Thus, choice is not imposed by
a prevailing or historical structure and system, but can be challenged
and criticized. There is more than one way to look at and respond to
individual and community mental health and mental illness and we
have to accept that prevailing ideologies will inevitably presume an
'accurate' view of the world. We also know that our realization of mental health promotion challenges the individualist, rational and mechanistic functions of a powerful system and the 'professionals' who work
in it.

The future role of the mental health worker within statutory provision is becoming more tenuous. There is an increasing pressure to
provide health and social care to people with enduring mental health
problems, and the standard vehicle for this is the community mental
health team (CMHT). This asylum model in community settings only

further distances relationships as partnerships and entrenches the role of mental health promotion as an adjunct to mental illness, not as a realization of community participation. Duplication of a dysfunctional perspective in a CMHT reveals a lack of awareness of alternative explanations and solutions and reduces interaction to mechanistic delivery. It also distances thinking as to the possibility of seeing mental health and its promotion as everybody's business. Key initiatives being developed include multidisciplinary outreach teams working seven days a week, twenty-four hours a day trying to maintain a comprehensive service to maintain people in the community. Education and training are important parts of this development identified by the work undertaken in high expressed emotion and psychosocial intervention, in line with the Health of the Nation's impetus in terms of tertiary approaches.

Having said this, we would ask you to consider where the present educational experience is. It is still centred around the individual in a social context, rather than a social context with individuals (citizens) in and created by it. We now not only have the problem of individual pathologizing, but also 'social pathologizing' (Prior 1993). This is reflected in the targeting approach to problems, which loses the Health for All principle of equity. Inequalities will not be addressed by focusing workers on a deprived locality and therapy as a consequence of this approach. It might also require the skills and intervention at the level of community work and community development approaches (Dalley 1996). This invariably means working with rather than on an estate and as such requires changes in thinking and practice regarding what we mean by multiprofessional or interagency input in terms of our mental health needs. By this we mean that at the level of community involvement all relevant individuals or agencies, such as the police, the housing department, leisure and recreation staff, architects, members of tenants' associations, to name but a few, work together in identifying and supporting grass-roots change. If there is to be a change in emphasis in mental health practice, then current thinking is that we address this primarily in the 'social domain' in relation to community participation and 'care', as being the core concern and focus for change and mutuality in relationships (Barker 1995).

Practice in the voluntary and private domains. Scope for involvement and education and training with 'professionals'

. . . Invite just one user representative on to a committee comprised of professionals . . . . Never pay service users. Expect them to attend regularly as the only unpaid people in a room full of salaried people. Then they will stop embarrassing you with their presence . . . . Perceptions alter when mental health workers see patients and ex-patients as experts. And if we are not experts in mental health and distress, why this lip-service to self-advocacy? (Lindow 1996)

Organizations such as MIND have perhaps become conscious and unconscious leaders in looking at community mental health in its widest sense. We have come a long way from historically limited roles and function within the voluntary sector, although the ideology inherent in the growth of the Charitable Organization Society is never far away. The notions of 'charity' and the 'undeserving' are still a major part of what the voluntary sector has to pick up, as more and more local authorities shed their responsibilities. A quest for professionalism in the sense of 'good practice' has to be contemplated within a much wider political spectrum that now determines the lives of people in many inner-city, rural and deprived areas of the country. Not surprisingly, entrenched positions often develop a perverse life of their own as people struggle with ideological approval in terms of securing continued government funding, economic constraints, differing perspectives, agendas, management structures, personal dynamics and goals.

The continued rise of the 'self-help' movement, in terms of specific groups of people whose needs cannot be met within mainstream service, has to some extent offset and made less visible the ways in which people are addressing their mental health needs. Changes, in terms of more centralized funding, have confused any notion of need and want, and policy implementation has all too often been as a backlash to failed therapy at statutory level (MIND 1995). This is now being addressed in many positive ways and exposure to voluntary and independent sectors can be a positive experience for people coming from statutory agencies. As part of the development of the mental health promotion group in Sheffield we were always looking for ways to network both locally and nationally. We consider this an under-developed aspect of mental health promotion and one that involves more than having numerous leaflets on the notice board of an acute psychiatric in-patient unit.

The voluntary and user sector, particularly MIND, offers a range of alternatives which can be more clearly identified as relating to the radical and humanistic perspectives previously discussed. MIND's vision goes beyond the preparation and socialization process which creates the mental health professional. The social context we inhabit, and therefore communicate, at all levels of involvement in our personal and working lives already affects and permeates our professional decision making and action. A world of inequality, power constructs and dynamic change provides us with a set of value judgements, ideas and constructs to orientate our professional and nonprofessional existence.

As a publication specifically for those who have experience of mental health services *OpenMind* is a very useful resource with which to gauge the current state feelings and opinions about mental health and illness. It is usually the 'recipients' of such provision who are often the best judges of what is going on at grass roots level. It would seem that the worlds of the professional and the 'user' clash so much in mainstream mental health provision that it is only by a process of radical education and exposure of the roots of the problem that we can begin to redress or 'undo' some wrongs (Lindow 1996). There is increasing literature which highlights how limited 'professional' expertise is in this field (Barham and Hayward 1995; Read and Reynolds 1996).

Professional input into voluntary and user-led service initiatives

The individual involved in the educational experience preparing for mental health practice does not come as a clean slate. He or she includes a collection of experiences, ideas and values which can inform MHP action. The advantages of such experiences are significant. Although some of them may be stereotypical and therefore potentially oppressive, many of the skills, competencies and styles of life apparent can be drawn upon to enrich the training and educational experience. This potential has been exploited positively within the voluntary sector. A focus on training has consistently maximized the skills and experiences of users, carers and survivors of mental illness and the systems and practices of psychiatry. The development of training for voluntary agencies, users and professionals in the legitimacy and practical application of support groups for 'voice hearers' is one contemporary example. Other training has included involving mental health teams, users and voluntary agencies to provide destigmatizing training in the school setting.

The advantages of such educational approaches include:

- Opportunities to invest and involve previously disempowered groups and individuals
- Legitimation of a process of participation, and resource and skill sharing
- Positive redefinition for practitioners and the voluntary sector of boundaries and roles
- Enablement of a broader picture of mental health to be examined and understood

The inclusion of the 'professional' in voluntary and user-led training is an important step in redirecting training and education into a wider context of learning experiences. If your course leaders or fellow students are able to acknowledge their own mental health needs and problems, it allows for more frank and practical debate. It also enables solutions to be debated and developed in a climate of recognizing difference and consensus. Within most educational and training elements of mental health practice, self-disclosure is now considered an essential element in redressing some of the boundaries which delineate 'felt' psychological experience from a label of mental illness. Obviously, once one enters into the statutory system it becomes increasingly hard to form alliances with the voluntary sector. Yet voluntary agencies have a major role to play in providing placement experience, and entering into contractual and curriculum obligations if interagency collaboration is the way forward. The voluntary sector provides a more positive forum where people from differing cultural and ethnic backgrounds can collaborate rather than be dominated by bureaucratic statutory agencies in the fight to challenge institutional racism and its negative practices (Ahmad 1990).

Concerns

One of the main problems facing voluntary agencies such as MIND is that in the current political and economic climate they are somehow expected to fulfil everyone's needs, primarily because this is a cost-effective way to offset the deficiencies within current statutory policies and practice. If 'shelter' can be found, because no one wants to be entered into statutory provision as it has developed, this detracts from the lack of the financial investment at central level so needed for dynamic mental health practice and the needs of individual people (DOH 1996, *Spectrum of Care*). At the same time, the continual need to tighten up a flawed Mental Health Act, as we discuss further in Chapter 9, dominates media and public perceptions and economic investment. This indicates that in the main the voluntary sector cannot impact at a strategic level of economic planning, except to highlight problem areas and raise the profile of their particular concerns where it can have most effect. There are additional problems when different agencies in the voluntary sector hold opposing beliefs about the cause of, say, schizophrenia, and this further confuses what priority is given to 'treatment' for many thousands of people who become subsumed under this label. As the internal market pares service contracts to the bone, it is unlikely that mental health promotion will take priority or that agencies will be capable of investing in new ideas, with demands for education and training being handled in a piecemeal and uncoordinated way (Dalley 1996). Dalley also points out that, in her opinion, in both voluntary and statutory provision 'there is an almost total absence of nonsexist options.

Few, if any, communal initiatives in the field of care provision operate on explicitly stated feminist principles' (p.145).

Private sector

In the private sector, by the very great problematic of making human distress a business venture, it is very difficult to identify what educational experiences there are and who and what they are determined by. There are very few private nursing homes for older people, for example, owned by nurses, profit being such a powerful primary motive in supporting conservative ideology. From our knowledge of some of the private provision for the mentally ill that we have encountered, or heard about, there is an assumption that paying untrained staff nearly half the suggested minimum wage is acceptable, while at the same time expecting enormous dedication and skill for which most are not trained. Then not providing adequate education and training can only compound the problems being faced in this sector. There are presumably many areas of 'good practice', and it is up to people to raise the profile of their service and also to be accountable to wider, not contracted, inspection mechanisms. Many people, especially the elderly mentally ill, are being forced to live in circumstances which perhaps provide the basic necessities but do little to enhance their mental health.

In such key areas as GP fundholding and the prison service there is continual movement to decentralize and make accountable, by using funding as the sole criterion for existence. Community mental health teams, as the heart of coordination of care in mental health practice, are subject to the particular requirements of individual trust managers and have had little chance to forge cooperative partnerships in the private and voluntary sectors. The requirements of care management have contracted rather than redefined needs assessment and this will be further highlighted in the next section.

User involvement/advocacy

> One great challenge for survivors is the establishment of our own identities. We are not only survivors of a mental health system that regularly fails to meet our wants and needs. We are also survivors of social attitudes and practices that exclude and discount our experience. Many of the identities society would have us assume – the mental patient, the vagabond, the tragic victim of disease – are ones we would never choose for ourselves. (Campbell 1993b)

We consider that the role of mental health promotion is pivotal in terms of both service users and workers involved with changing much of current psychiatric/mental health practice into a more empowering and equitable process. The rationale for the development of Direct Power, for example, is much welcomed and hopefully will be used by professionals to enhance care management approaches (Leader 1995). We know in our locality that multiple packs have been bought by managers for staff to use in various mental health settings. This is at least a start, and we would hope that in other parts of the country this is being repeated. In the words of the groups and individuals who contributed to the pack, the 'system' must be failing a lot of people to highlight so many key areas of concern. We have highlighted part of the rationale outlined at the beginning of direct power.

Box 5.1 **Community Support Network and Brixton Community Sanctuary believe that:**

- Individuals are unique
- They are of unlimited worth
- They have the right to the means and resources which enable them to live a full life in the community
- They have the right to self-determination and to be able to develop a support network that is tailored to their individual needs
- They have the right to be consulted with and to participate in the planning, management and development of local services

In our collective experience, people refuse to take up services because in their experience they found that services and professionals:

- are oppressive and controlling
- see them as problems to be solved, filed and dispatched rather than human beings in need of dignity, respect and consideration
- crush individualism
- emphasize the needs and political agendas of those in charge of the services and the workers
- deny the people the right of citizenship
- promote dependency and the 'sick' role
- are not directly accountable to users
- marginalize people's natural support networks and
- devalue people's experiences and feelings

The *Direct Power* pack provides those needing mental health services with a chance to develop their own personal profile/care/action plan and partnership agreement from a user-led perspective. Hopefully it is the way forward in offsetting the limiting use of written accounts, as in care plans and legal documentation by statutory workers, and will be taken up by them in determining a different emphasis on need assessment. This creative account is also emphasized in one of the latest DOH documents *Building Bridges* (DOH 1995e), but it is addressed in relation to people considered to have serious and enduring mental health problems where the chance of this taking priority over assessment of risk and dangerousness is obvious in the current climate.

In MIND's recent publication on reshaping the future for community mental health care, they identify clearly the tenuous relationship between need and want in identifying how the needs of the 'whole person' might be better met. (See Boxes 5.2 and 5.3.)

Box 5.2 **MIND'S criteria**

NEED =
Mind – in line with the disabled living movement – believes that the right and opportunity to live independently and equally with others is the starting point for a user-centred approach to needs assessment.

Need as defined by doctors tends to be tied to strict diagnostic categories.

WANT=
[Want] as defined by service users draws attention to ordinary human experience rather than medical labels and may be more conducive to developing a user-centred assessment process. It deals with what is useful to every individual and enables people to match up their aspirations and ambitions with their care plan and the services on offer. The possibility for achievement encourages greater self-esteem and self-empowerment, and allows ordinary local resources to be brought into consideration as ways of improving quality of life for users. Above all, a user-centred assessment process increases informed consent and choice, by providing users with a greater say in decision-making.

Box 5.3 **Reshaping the future. MIND's twelve core components: Fulfilling the needs of the whole person**

1. Opportunities for achieving life quality
2. Personal support during the period of distress
3. Support during a personal crisis
4. Practical help at home
5. Opportunities to assure income
6. Somewhere to live or stay
7. Access to paid or unpaid occupation
8. Access to information that supports fair treatment
9. Someone to talk to

10. Opportunities for assuring mobility and travel
11. Ways of improving access to and contact with services
12. Opportunities for taking a break.

Reshaping the Future: MIND's Policy for Community Mental Health Care
(MIND 1995)

The emphasis from this perspective is immediately more positive and more focused on the service-user. The questions that people would then need to ask themselves would, in terms of self-assessment and profiling, be from a different perspective, i.e. What words do you use to describe the unique person that you are?, What would you describe as your strengths?, What do you do well?, What things would you like to learn?, Are there things you would like to improve? Obviously, these could be just words without the necessary attitudes and values needed to underpin mutual care relationships from this perspective. This requires a forum about a 'common' language that is needed to replace dominant psychiatric 'jargon'. Education and training are vital in this area, where the views and opinions of service users still need a higher profile to counter the deficiencies and power imbalances inherent in the world of the professionals and the state. Pavilion Publishing have a wide range of training material, including one specifically identifying 'dual-needs', for people with a learning disability and mental health problems. Within current nursing and social work journals there seems to be a realistic understanding of how difficult and painful changes on this scale might be (Dalrymple and Burke 1995; Rudman 1996). Combined with a real crisis in community/mental health nursing, the move to practices that are built on a more cooperative 'paradigm' would mean a dramatic reappraisal of everything that has gone before. Rudman sought the opinions of a number of users to incorporate their views in the development of a curriculum for mental health nursing. He also collated some emerging themes that would support the elements for a framework for MHP we have identified. We reproduce these themes in Table 5.1 as a point of discussion.

Table 5.1 **User's views identified as 'themes' in Rudman's Study**	**Knowledge**	**Skills**	**Qualities**
	Individual differences	Counselling/ meaningful dialogue	Caring
	Avoiding narrowness	Sensitivity to nonverbal cues	Maintaining caring despite socialization
(continued opposite)	Understanding, not labelling behaviour	Accepting people's experiences	Approachability, immediacy and presence

Knowledge	Skills	Qualities	Table 5.1 **User's views identified as 'themes' in Rudman's Study** (*continued*)
Knowledge of life/ maturity, local areas and resources, effects of hospitalization and physical care	Inspiring confidence, avoiding jargon and stereotyped responses; giving information openly; continuity of support; renouncing one's own worries; ability to take control when needed; sensitive defusing of tense situations	Professional demeanour	

Rudman (1996), p.197

There seems to be a positive development taking place within the user movement that has strong links to the role of the advocate in mental health practice. In certain parts of the country user-development workers provide a role that can support not only service users but also nurses and social workers at the interface of the purchaser/provider split. Identified ways are now being considered that could mean a much broader investment into user organizations and would require a different focus to education and training. One initiative, discussed in a 1996 edition of community care, uses employed workers, who are funded by purchasers, with a brief to collect and collate views that support the way grants are funded. Also, development workers and users work together to help local user groups develop links and secure services and identify components for formal research projects. This process seems to mirror the need for professionals to have experience of community development in the way we have considered in terms of playing an active role in MHP.

Advocacy

> The illusion of power over the feelings of others is a deadly chimera . . . .
> There are few people in my life now who have the real political power to
> impose close-quarter tyranny on my actions. (Kopp 1974, p.64)

More recently there has been great interest in advocacy, within both nursing and social work. The role of advocate was clearly defined in Peplau's model for psychiatric nursing, as early as the 1950s, and there is an acute need, for those who have most contact with people experiencing mental illness, to act on their behalf and carry out their wishes (Jones 1996). Whether this role is a tenable one within mainstream provision requires further evaluation, but is increasingly considered as integral to the effective functioning of community mental health teams (Tudor 1996). The concept of citizen advocacy has strong links to the development of rights and charters, as identified by Dalrymple and Burke (1995) in their book, and to the development of legal advocacy to support those having to fight for both legal and civil recognition. From the opinions we have sought from those working and training in this aspect of service provision, utilizing advocacy services is considered of paramount importance, especially in supporting black people in their tenuous position in psychiatric theory and practice.

Community as a setting, a resource and underpinning social participation

> Human reality is messy and ambiguous – and so moral decisions, unlike abstract ethical principles, are ambivalent. It is in this sort of world that we must live, and yet, as if defying the worried philosophers who cannot conceive of an 'unprincipled' morality, a morality without foundations, we demonstrate day by day that we can live, or learn to live, or manage to live in such a world, though few of us would be ready to spell out, if asked, what the principles that guide us are, and fewer still would have heard about the 'foundations' which we allegedly cannot do without to be good and kind to each other. (Bauman 1993, p.32)

We consider that community education and development have a vital role to play in mental health promotion and accept that this always has to be put into context with the conflicting nature of welfare provision. Community work, for example, since its inception as a strategic route for the maintenance of dominant conservative values, quickly fell into disrepute when the community development programmes of the 1950s and 1960s became too radical and too successful, especially in inner-city areas and in highlighting gross inequality in Britain (Craig *et al.* 1982). Its reification as a core element of health and social care practice is fragmented, and as ever tied to economic necessity and ideology. As the blurring of health and social care provision becomes a major factor in continued welfare provision, the 'community' is now the 'milieu' in which this is enacted and it is apparent that many people are not equipped to cope in this predominately social world.

Having begun with the premise that mental health is inextricably linked to cultural-socio-economic factors, it might be useful to reconsider the starting point of community work education and training in its many forms, and how applicable this still is in envisaging the level of community involvement required in mental health promotion. As long ago as 1968, the Calouste Gulbenkian Foundation published their report on community work. It saw its remit as being:

> . . . essentially concerned with affecting the course of social change through the two processes of analysing social situations and forming relationships

with different groups to bring abut some desirable change. It has three main aims: the first is to the democratic process of involving people in thinking, deciding, planning and playing an active part in the development and operation of services that affect their daily lives; the second relates to the value for personal fulfilment of belonging in a community; the third is concerned with the need in community planning to think of actual people in relation to other people and the satisfaction of their needs as persons, rather than to focus attention upon a series of separate needs and problems. This means working within constant tensions between people's needs and the scarce resources available to meet them, between conflicting demands of different groups, and different ideas about the kind of change that is desirable. Organizational structures and administration are also important in impeding or facilitating these purposes.

Community work is only one aspect of the far broader issue of how to meet people's needs and give them an effective say in what these are and how they want them met. It is part of a protest against apathy and complacency and against distant and anonymous authority. It is also part of the whole dilemma of how to reconcile the 'revolution of human dissent' with the large scale organisation and economic and social planning which seem to be inseparably interwoven with the parallel revolution of rising expectations. This boils down to the problem of how to give meaning to democracy. Obviously many people are trying to do this in many ways. The question for community work is whether organisational structures can be devised and people trained and employed to facilitate citizen participation and to make it more effective, as well as making public and voluntary services more acceptable and usable. In short, community work is a means of giving life to local democracy. (Calouste Gulbenkian Foundation 1968)

Whatever aspect of 'community' is being addressed by health and social care workers, the importance and relevance of people living in any given environment cannot be ignored in terms the above. The limitations of community mental health teams and the continuing difficulties with assessing the role and function of community psychiatric nurses and social workers are nowhere near being resolved (Brooker *et al.* 1996). What we do know is that these issues are becoming more sharply focused as the need for services for those with serious or enduring mental health problems overshadows the needs of others such as older adults and those with multiple and complex needs such as those who have learning disabilities and mental health problems. If mental health promotion has any strategic value, it is important that whatever meaning is attached to 'community', be this community provision, community care, community participation and community development, a primary consideration should be to identify the roles involved in this and to encourage practice which overcomes the boundaries of 'professional' status and is the catalyst for meaningful action. It is obviously very important to have knowledge about, or even

> Consider this account. What has happened to affect our commitment to community democracy and citizen participation, apart from the national lottery?

access to, the vast amount of literature on the subject of 'community' and to come to know and assess this in its many forms and guises. If, as it is recognized, that knowledge can equate to power and increased autonomy for clients experiencing mental health problems, why do we not practise what we preach? What factors prevent this? A limited vision will provide limited accounts and resources and action. Perhaps nurses and social workers interested in mental health promotion, in terms of community participation, will feel they have to be all things to all people. Primarily they should at least be able to relate to fellow human beings, and be able to identify with them in a more open and honest climate about health and illness needs and why they hold the beliefs they do. That is preferable to having to listen to professionals glibly using terms like the 'worried well' while at the same time ignoring the determinant position of themselves and others in any given community, neighbourhood area, or society (Amies 1996).

Sheffield's contribution and its relevance to education and training

In Chapter 1 we highlighted a research study published in Sheffield which attempted to give an account of the development of MHP in our locality. This was achieved by the use of a postal questionnaire sent out to all GPs citywide by the FHSA, and also included as many people and professionals who had active involvement in mental health provision. The survey confirmed that there is a lack of research and development in this field and that this is an important factor in determining appropriate educational and training initiatives. We have reproduced in Chapter 10 some of the responses from the survey and the development of the Mental Health Promotion Group in which we were involved (Monach and Spriggs 1995).

The researchers found that of the total correspondents in their survey, only a quarter, 'saw themselves as having a lead role or specialist interest in MHP'. The group most likely to make this claim was that of community workers. In terms of the extent of training in MHP, both 'experienced' and 'initiated', two-thirds did not consider that they had experienced any such initiatives. An identified dilemma was the specific need of key organizations, such as the housing department, for staff training about mental health and illness. Was this a key role for the MHP worker to fulfil in an *ad hoc* approach to the problem? Or was it a failure at the level of communication between agencies to meet specific targets in relation to MHP which created the problem in the first place? This is a key problematic, given the vast network of services that exist and the vested interests of each. We again point out that in our initial definition or premise this conflict, and the process of managing it, is a core element of our practice.

The role of the mental health promotion worker has developed, as outlined in Chapter 1, increasingly in terms of a strategic role at the interface of the purchaser/provider divide. Further research and development are vital and we again highlight some areas for this in Chapter 10. We had hoped to refine the questionnaires developed by Monach and Spriggs so they were applicable to evaluating the work we had initiated with health and social care educationalists, practitioners and students. Although our involvement in the mental health branch programme courses for Project 2000 was limited, because of other teaching and work commitments, it did provide enormous scope for assessing mental health promotion as a core element of mental health practice. At times this process again raised expectations that we could not fulfil. The attempt to introduce anti-oppressive practice as underpinning any care practices we were engaged in caused many heated debates. This was experienced in the classroom with students, in challenging strongly held oppressive attitudes and assumptions. At a wider level, it was seen in changing our School of Nursing policy to incorporate this difference in emphasis in the light of the limitations of merely stating equal opportunity policies and expecting everything else to fall into place or to carry on just as before.

Conclusions

In this chapter we have re-examined the core problematic of addressing mental health promotion in terms of the public, professionals and the state. We have considered the foundational nature of such practice and how important theoretical accounts might or might not be in focusing our attention on the specific psycho-socio-economic-cultural variants which should enhance our understanding of mental health and illness. We are concerned that with all the information and knowledge available to us, it is still all too often realized in entrenched Eurocentric ideas and the language of 'professionals' within psychiatric or mental health practice. We highlighted a philosophy of education in terms of radical practice, as envisaged by Friere and developed by other theorists in relation to our health needs. Consideration of primary health care strategies is essential in any discussion about mental health promotion, and has strong links to our desire for more equitable community participation. We identified the emerging role of the voluntary and private sectors in taking over many of the functions of statutory provision and redressing many of the wrongs being done to people because of misplaced ideas about what constitutes 'care' and 'therapy'. Many more individuals are turning to counselling within voluntary and private settings both to avoid marginalization of their problems and to get away from the excesses of medication and 'treatment' of their identity, risk and dangerousness rather than their problems! We have determined that what is lacking in education and training initiatives in this field is an ability to grasp the very nature of mental health promotion. Much more research and development are needed to determine where we should invest and prioritize in terms of collaborative care. Reaching for some 'moral high ground', while at the same time ignoring the obvious, is not a healthy relationship between individuals whom we identified in terms of the public, professionals and the state.

We know that our identification of anti-oppressive practice as being the linchpin of our framework will have limited appeal to people who want a quick result either by some 'scientifically' proved specification of 'a mentally healthy person', or a short training course which can show that this aspect is being addressed so that everyone can go away with the handouts and communicate in the language of 'been there, seen it, done that'! Our idea is that one has to be humbled first. You have to address your own position as oppressed and oppressor and accept that although some people might accept your definitions and your approach, others might not. It does mean that it can take a long time to reach these goals:

- To feel secure enough about oneself to discuss these issues
- To be in the right environment to do so
- To accept one's racist or prejudicial assumptions and understand why some black people think that some white people cannot do so
- To accept that two wrongs do not make a right
- To become aware of the full extent of oppression and not to have negated one's own position in it as being less or more important than others
- By learning in the right environment, to accept difference, not to fear it

In our work in education and practice in mental health we have considered the many ways in which learning takes place. One way we have found that has great 'power' and the ability to facilitate dialogue and ownership of feelings and values is through the very wise words that, mostly, one has to attribute to others but which occasionally come forth from oneself! The reawakening of 'oral history', 'story telling' and 'wise words' is considered to be an integral part of how we involve ourselves in the promotion of our mental health. It is very often by word of mouth, and translation by 'the public' of 'the experts'' words and actions, that people manage to relate to one another. This spans educational texts, literature, music, and the media. We are all in some kind of 'melting pot' in terms of race, gender and class, and in the late twentieth century the message by which oppressions are both perpetuated and highlighted takes many forms. We have said that mental health is a double-edged sword if we do not accept that our life is fraught with paradoxes and dilemmas, which are usually not resolved by the present educational experience of the 'masses', the more traditional 'therapies', medication, or dependency. Alleviation of distress is only part of what mental health promotion is about. There is no easy route *to saying what you mean and meaning what you say*, and it is obvious that we need a different platform from which to do so.

6 From theory to practice – prevention and education

Any new venture in the field of preventive work in mental health must take as its central task the transformation of passive receivers of mental health services into active participants in the understanding and the solutions to their own and their neighbours' distress. (Holland 1992)

Mental health education can develop both the capacities of people to achieve mental heath, and also increase knowledge about the environmental determinants of mental and social health and the skills to campaign for changes. (Tilford 1995)

Key themes:
- Prevention
- Education
- Professional contribution

Overview

This chapter examines mental health promotion at primary, secondary and tertiary levels and identifies the strengths and weakness such a model can provide. We begin with an introduction to the concept of prevention and examine education in the mental health and illness field. We would stress that what is most important is to delineate boundaries, in terms of the primary, secondary and tertiary split, only when it is necessary, and to bear in mind the need for a pragmatic approach to a framework for practice. This basis of what could be termed 'holistic' practice is relevant in any consideration of current approaches to mental health care, and is seen as underpinning the health and social care needs of the 'whole' person. Examples highlighted give a picture of key aspects which are currently being addressed at the level of human response, policy, practice and research.

Definitions

The definition most familiar to practitioners, and one frequently cited, is that devised by Caplan (1961), with a distinction between three levels of prevention: primary, secondary and tertiary. More recently, Rogers and

Pilgrim (1996), describe these three aspects of prevention as primary prevention relating to a focus on structures and processes as 'psychotoxic' life events and precipitating factors: secondary prevention as accurate screening – with a policy focus on primary care as the setting and vehicle for this; and tertiary prevention as minimizing the impact of illness and preventing relapse. These definitions and possible interventions from a mental illness perspective are expanded in Table 6.1.

Table 6.1
Levels of prevention and interventions

Primary	Secondary ✓	Tertiary
Prevention: The process involved in reducing the risk that people in the community will become ill with a mental illness	**Prevention:** The activities involved in reducing the duration of established cases of mental illness	**Prevention:** The prevention of what Caplan (1961) called 'defect and crippling' among the members of a community
Practice: Anticipating and pre-empting disease occurrence. Targeting of vulnerable groups	**Practice:** Intervening at an early stage in disease causation and/or occurrence. This is the realm of hospital and community services to promptly treat and reduce a deterioration of a mental illness condition	**Practice:** Preventing relapse or minimizing subsequent impairment. This centres around the prevention and treatment of long-term mental illness, such as behavioural and coping strategies for families supporting people with schizophrenia
Interventions	**Interventions**	**Interventions**
• Public education on social and psychological aspects of mental ill-health • Identification of at-risk groups • Information and support to at-risk groups • Advice and counselling • Monitoring effectiveness of action	• Rapid response • Home assessment and treatment • Crisis intervention • Continuity of care • Education and support to carers • Personal coping strategies	• Anti-discrimination in health care of people with mental illness • Coping strategies for carers and people with enduring physical and mental illness • Respite care • Liaison psychiatry – sharing skills with other health and social care services

This three-level approach to prevention is also emphasized in the Mental Health Nursing Review (see Chapter 2). To meet the recommendations, liaison work between community mental health nurses and other members of the primary health care team is called for. Primary care is identified as a key setting for prevention and vulnerability as a determining factor in targeting activity in this model as set out in Table 6.2.

Table 6.2
A suggested framework for collaborative working by nurses, midwives and health visitors in mental health care

Location	Activity
Primary prevention: Reducing the incidence of mental illness.	Work with vulnerable people or those at risk of mental illness.
Health visitors, district nurses, specialist nurses, practice nurses and the specialist support of the mental health nurse.	
Secondary prevention: Early detection leading to prompt intervention.	Early detection and case finding, leading to early intervention. Work mostly carried out in the primary health care setting.
As above only 'requires continuous liaison and some casework by mental health nurse.	
Tertiary prevention: Treatment and active intervention with established mental illness.	Early intervention, effective treatment and rehabilitation requiring active case management.
Mental health nurses in hospitals, residential, day and community care. Liaison with nurses in the above categories.	

The three-element model is also drawn upon by the Faculty of Public Health Medicine (1996) in a publication on commissioning district mental health services. It states (p.29) that

> The evidence for effectiveness of primary prevention of mental health problems such as public education, improving social conditions and specific targeting of high-risk groups requires further research. However, specific secondary and tertiary prevention, that is the prevention of social disablement through early identification and treatment, is possible.

This rather narrow view is one we would not endorse. While research and evaluation are to be encouraged, the need for prevention of the onset or manifestation of a mental illness is desirable. This is particularly the case in the area of suicide.

Is this model familiar to your practice?

How will it deal with people who do not have acute or enduring mental health problems?

Suicide and prevention

One very important and central concern of mental health care is how suicide is addressed in terms of preventive work. Suicide is seen as a major cause of preventable death. Figures for July 1994 (Williams and Morgan 1994) give 5542 known cases in England. This is higher than the figure for road traffic accidents and fails to take account of the sensitivity of the issue, which results in many suicides being recorded as accidental death. As a key target (C3) in the Health of the Nation, suicide has been highlighted in government strategy and policy as an area to be addressed.

Williams and Morgan (1994), in a thematic review of suicide prevention, suggest a range of guidance and state that 'Suicide is not always preventable, but sound clinical practice can help avert it in certain clinical situations' (p.5). Such honesty in the field of prevention is welcome and demonstrates the complex nature of the problem. However, we would point out that more than clinical practices are required if it is to be realistically addressed. This is of even more importance given that the population that the Health of the Nation target refers to – the severely mentally ill. Although often surrounded by a range of clinical expertise, they are a group for whom often that may be the only human contact they have. If these issues are not to be addressed and solutions to them found, then targets, as relevant as they are to clinical staff, cannot hope to be achieved.

Appleby and Araya (1991) see suicide from a public health perspective or as an outcome measure in the evaluation of psychiatric services. The reality is that the two overlap. Appleby describes four elements of a suicide prevention programme (Box 6.1). For a more detailed approach, the Health Advisory Service (HAS) gives a range of training and intervention points to deal with suicide prevention.

Box 6.1 **Appleby's four elements of a suicide prevention programme**

1. Identification of risk factors and preventive influences in high-risk groups
2. Early detection of persons at risk
3. Adequate preventive pathways
4. Suicide monitoring.

As part of a more general critique which includes suicide as one aspect, Hosman and Veltman (1994) see prevention as closely related to rising costs in the health sector and consider that this deflects the focus onto the application of financial and economic concepts and management practices such as audit, quality, cost-effectiveness and efficiency. It is within this context that current approaches to prevention in health and illness can become entrenched. Hosman and Veltman gathered a range of information on the effectiveness of health promotion and health interventions and the quality of the evaluation of research and

Do you feel that the three-level model is sufficient in preventing suicide, or are actions wider than health interventions required?

outcomes. The objective was to improve the accessibility of information on the effectiveness of health education/promotion. The review consisted of a set of criteria drawn up for analysing published studies. The results reveal, perhaps most crucially to policy makers and funders of services, that there are demonstratable long-term positive effects in terms of health and social and economic gain.

Four elements of prevention

Finally, Downie, Fyfe and Tannahill (1990) highlight the deficiencies of the traditional primary, secondary and tertiary definition of prevention. Instead they suggest that the focus should span four elements. This moves away from a disease model to a more dynamic approach to prevention as one part of a model for promoting health (Box 6.2).

Box 6.2 **Four 'foci' for prevention**

1. Prevention of the onset or first manifestation of a disease process, or some other first occurrence, through risk reduction; for example, coping strategies for dealing with stress and depression

2. Prevention of the progression of a disease process or other unwanted state, through early detection when this favourably affects outcome; for example, early detection of depression in primary care

3. Prevention of avoidable complications of an irreversible, manifest disease or some other unwanted state; for example, prevention of further complications associated with depression such as homelessness or debt

4. Prevention of the recurrence of an illness or other unwanted phenomenon; for example, prevention of a further episode of depression.

How then have some of these models been developed in practice? We will start with an examination of the work of Newton.

Is the traditional approach to prevention at variance with the broader health-promotion approach we suggest? Or can it be accommodated into a package of measures and methods which look at health as well as illness?

Prevention and mental illness

Newton (1988) in *Preventing Mental Illness* highlights three areas to address:

1. Targeting vulnerable individuals, which Newton describes as the medical model for prevention
2. Helping people to take control over their own lives
3. Making maximum use of natural, voluntary and community support networks.

This is contrasted with the health promotion model which is described as one which 'targets the general population with measures known to be preventive of disorder for a few and assumed to be health-promoting for the rest. Mental health promotion methods include communication, education, legislation, fiscal measures, organizational change and community development' (Newton 1988).

In elaborating a model for prevention, she describes the 'disease model' approach. This takes into account the historical precedent of introducing preventive measures prior to the aetiology of disorder being completely understood. In our argument, we would also state that from this approach, biological or genetic determinants of mental illness are not major factors. Despite the advance of psychotropic medication for stabilizing and ameliorating the impact of illness, it is the social and economic consequences of mental ill-health which are of importance for sufferer, carer and community alike.

Another approach identified by Newton is a health perspective as opposed to an illness perspective in relation to prevention: helping people who are not ill to remain free of illness. Just as there is a range of underlying factors which may increase the likelihood of ill-health, especially mental health, there are significant numbers of the population who remain symptom free. There is also the issue of oppression, discrimination and other factors that result in people being unable or unwilling to use services in the first place. In the case of the government's response to health and social care and the shift to rationing, there are also implications in terms of populations and illnesses that are deemed of greater importance than others. Thus, we have the shift to the preventive elements of severe mental illness such as schizophrenia, which focuses on psychosocial and behavioural competence building, and which have status placed upon them and resources allocated to them.

Community-orientated and population-wide approaches to health and prevention have never had the necessary resources, nor have they been properly evaluated to determine their effectiveness. One of the strengths of the new behavioural–cognitive paradigm in treating severe mental illness is that it may reveal more explicitly the effectiveness of interventions.

The health model of prevention is aimed at the population as a whole, something in keeping with a health promotion philosophy. Newton's review of the model highlights factors found among the healthy population which are presumed to counterbalance damaging external influences. Recurring examples of protective factors include knowledge, economic security, coping skills and support.

Newton elaborates her ideas in a second work, *Preventing Mental Illness in Practice* (1992). In this account she accepts that preventive work does not result in immediate or short-term results in the way that clinical work with service users can. Newton is also explicit about the concept of prevention in terms of it consisting of action focused at people who are not defined as 'cases' – that is individuals whose symptoms and experience have not led them to specialist mental illness services.

Prevention issues: examples

In the case of practitioners, the area of stress is significant for professional and associated workers in treatment and care. Cozens and Firth (1994) use longitudinal data to make recommendations to employers, educators and professional bodies on ways to improve the mental health of doctors and to explore ways to identify those at risk as students. At a broader workplace level, two documents relate to this area of prevention and education. The first is: *The Health of the Nation: ABC of Mental Health in the Workplace. A Resource Pack for Employers* (DOH 1995f). The pack consists of eleven fact sheets which summarize key points about mental health for employers. It covers the following areas:

- Why do I need to know about mental health?
- What is a mental health problem?
- How can I recognize mental health problems?
- What causes mental health problems?
- What can I do about it?
- How can I help prevent problems developing?
- What if a problem has developed?
- Recruitment issues/return to work
- What is a health policy? (Mental health components)
- Sources of help
- Publication list

Good practice example: HEA and multimedia

Leonard (1994) identifies possible future information technology (IT) developments for health services, including patient information and education, resource production in professional and medical training, patients records, health data and audit. Examples of applying IT include interactive video programmes for cancer patients and their families at home, a depression information programme and a cancer information service which use touch-screen technology for use in public sites such as libraries and GPs' surgeries.

Health of the Nation

According to the Key Area Handbook: Mental Illness (DOH 1993a) the following fall into primary prevention as part of promoting mental health:

- Social isolation: support from friends, family and other support structures
- Living conditions: homelessness or inadequate housing
- Sensory or physical impairment: reducing the additional risk of disabling depression
- Child abuse: the early detection and management of emotional and physical abuse
- Awareness of mental health: increasing people's ability to recognize their own stress and look after themselves

Such a list of possible primary preventive action begs the question asked by Monach and Spriggs (1995) when examining definitions of mental health: 'Is it about personal change or social change? Life skills training or social action? Personal adjustment or empowerment?' (p.6). A purely preventive approach appears to squeeze out consideration of the significant social factors which underpin, or undermine, our potential for mental health. In order to expand upon prevention, we will now look at the field of education and attempt to develop a synthesis for practice between preventive and educative approaches to the promotion of mental health.

Education

Health education is communication actively aimed at enhancing positive health and preventing or diminishing ill-health in individuals and groups, through influencing the beliefs, attitudes, and behaviour of those with power and the community at large. (Downie *et al.* 1990)

The role of education and educational strategies is significant for MHP. The issue of information and education has been raised by users, professionals and policy makers alike; but it is not a quick fix. With educational methods can come sets of values and approaches that can

What are the implications of the new technology for preventive approaches to mental health issues?

Does the Internet and use of computer technology offer opportunities for users, self-help groups and professionals?

be more damaging than they are health-promoting. As the approach to health of Downie will testify, education is an overlapping sphere of activity which lies at the heart of a health-promoting approach, but, without preventive and protective elements it is too narrow an approach. The focus for the professional services has always centred around primary and secondary approaches.

Models of health education

There are essentially four models of education: (1) a traditional behaviour change model which has strong connections with medicine and an underlying principle of orthodoxy; (2) an educational model with a focus on choice; (3) a self-empowerment model emphasizing autonomy; (4) a radical–collective action model taking a social change approach. It is worth examining the key features of these models to identify possible interventions for MHP. The models are compared in Table 6.3.

Tilford (1995) describes the 'embedded approach' regarding the way mental health education is part of all other programmes and approaches. She recommends epidemiological data, social indicators and community-based needs assessment as subjective and objective measures for programme planning and implementation in this area.

Tilford argues that the structural determinants of mental health need to be addressed in parallel: an educational strategy alone will not suffice. We could then consider the appropriateness of a settings approach to MHP, e.g. in schools and hospitals. This also suggests a health promotion rather than a health education approach to the issue of mental health and mental illness antistigma work. Although we aim at normalizing and humanizing mental illness and the myths surrounding it, there is much that perhaps should not be humanized: the abuses within and outside of psychiatry in the shape of physical and other treatments.

The prevention and education movement has a long history in the mental illness area and can be viewed, according to the Clifford Beers Foundation (1996), in the following chronology. There is inevitable overlap with the development of health policy and public health and health promotion as outlined in Chapter 2.

- **The European Reform Movement:** Action against child labour, women's rights movement and public health. This also resulted in better living conditions for mental patients in institutions.
- **The Mental Hygiene Movement** and the development of concepts of primary, secondary and tertiary prevention.
- **The World Federation for Mental Health:** The post-Second World War period saw a focus on prevention/education work with children

Looking at these four models which one would you say is the most appropriate for promoting mental health and why?

Table 6.3
Four models of education

	Traditional	Educational	Self-empowerment	Radical–collective action
Aims	To prevent ill-health by promoting behaviour change in individuals by compulsion or persuasion	To provide access to knowledge and resources to promote understanding and reasoning	To enhance self-concept, foster decision-making skills and develop interpersonal relationships	To encourage respect for self and others, group problem solving and critical social analysis awareness
Educator's role	Expert controlling the transmission of knowledge	Arbitrator exemplifying rational decision making	Facilitator to promote self-awareness	Energizer negotiating boundaries
Educated role	Passive, conforming, assimilating knowledge	Involved, negotiation of content, active participation	Active and interactive; individuals' behaviour and learning processes become the content	Active, collaborative, negotiating content and process; commitment to shared projects
Methods and approaches	Provision of information to raise awareness and reinforce predetermined behaviours. Use of posters, leaflets, advice sessions, lectures, demonstrations and texts	Discussion of information, analysis and synthesis. Use of debates, checklists, case studies, projects, games, trigger films	Provide individual and group settings to permit self-disclosure, reflection and encourage feedback. Includes counselling, role play, case study, reflective writing, art	Analysis of social situations and issues, recognition of power relationships and developing community skills. Includes media studies, community projects, action research, group discussions, community art
Evaluation	Recall of knowledge, behaviour change, illness prevented, reduced mortality and morbidity, safety and familiarity of methods	A range of achievements valued in relation to individual progress	Personal perceptions and evidence of personal growth and development	Increased sharing of responsibility and decision making, visible and public
Advantages	Efficient transmission of knowledge, efficient use of expertise, aims easily communicated and monitored	Varied methods increase likelihood of involvement; values people's contributions, encourages application of knowledge, transferable skills	Based on personal experience, values the individual; values development of self-esteem and group development	Conscientization; groups connect with relevant issues, mobilizes individual contributions and group support
Disadvantages	Dependency on educator or resistance, ignores individual differences, can be blame-inducing	Can be time-consuming; educator needs training and support	Risk taking, overintrusive, isolates skill learning from real-life contexts	Time-consuming and lengthy planning; can be manipulative

to forestall adult mental illness and with adults for the prevention of readmission of adults to hospital.

- **The 1960s and 1970s** saw developments such as personal growth, sex education, improvement in the socioeconomic position of women, mental health at work, the recognition of the impact of social class differences, access to care services, democratization of psychiatry, development of self-help and patient organizations.
- **The 1980s and 1990s** have seen a scientific approach to MHP. This is the rationale for the traditional services, but health promotion operates within a different arena. It remains focused within the social realm while still being located as a professional (emerging) discipline attempting to straddle both the statutory social policy and mainstream agencies and community development and empowerment. Key areas in the prevention field include work with children as young carers, the effects of divorce on family life and the individuals within it, strategies for adults in stress management and assertiveness approaches, mental health of refugees, depression, and eating disorders.

A review of the literature by Hosman and Veltman (1994) gives a sense of the breadth of opportunities for a range of agencies and organizations to engage in:

Individual counselling	Management consultancy
Early treatment	Network development
Group education	Development of new services
Consultation to primary care and community leaders	Social advocacy and social action
Training programmes	Human rights
Development and improvement of support systems	Legislation and political measures
Mass media education	

Most of the programmes reviewed came from the United States. Although Hosman and Veltman see mental health promotion and preventive education as one and the same, this view depends upon the interventions not only proving successful in the reduction of psychological problems and symptoms but in the longer-term benefits. The real difference between MHP and education is that the latter sees the outcomes in terms of reduction or removal of symptoms of mental ill-health. Thus, a programme for children of divorcees deals with behaving appropriately in terms of social interaction, but there is not enough acceptance of the very 'normal' response to loss of relationships and security. Mental health promotion has to span the practice of statutory provision and the folklore of how dealing with situations ranging from complete insanity to the inability of two people or families live with each other or next door to each other. The impact of racism and oppression on our mental health is highlighted both as a cause which could be prevented, education being a major determinant in this, and as a reaction to the complexity and paradox inherent in the human condition. This is something which mental health promotion can address without there being a means to an end, as there all too often is in mainstream psychiatric practice.

Synthesis

How then can the strengths of preventive and educative models of practice be drawn together within a mental health promotion framework? One way is through adoption of the model of overlapping spheres of prevention, education and protection as proposed by Downie *et al.*:

> Health promotion comprises efforts to enhance positive health and prevent ill-health, through the overlapping spheres of health education, prevention, and health protection. (Downie *et al.* 1990)

Another is to utilize the primary–secondary–tertiary model and adapt it to a wider approach – a mental health-promoting approach. This has been successfully achieved by the Trent Health Gain Investment Programme on Mental Health Promotion (HGIP 1994). Examples are given in Table 6.4. What this demonstrates is that preventive and educative approaches can be combined.

Table 6.4
Mental health promotion and mental illness prevention: concepts, strategies and examples (adopted from HGIP 1994)

Primary prevention

Mental health promotion

'The promotion of mental health is not solely for the purpose of disease prevention. It is to improve the quality of life for the whole population at all stages during their life.'[1]

Examples of proactive universal interventions

The Greater Easterhouse Mental Health Pilot Project, whose Education Working Group proposed a piece of research and evaluation around the impact of a play, aimed 'to correct erroneous ideas and attitudes previously held'.[2]

Secondary prevention

The Northampton Mental Health Project, one of the aims of which was 'to explain what community care means, how lay people can themselves play a part and why, from the medical point of view, it is important that they should do so.'[5]

Adult education course, in which the public spent structured times on the wards of a psychiatric hospital with discussion and support groups facilitated by medical and nursing staff.[6]

(*continued overleaf*)

Table 6.4 **Mental health promotion and mental illness prevention: concepts, strategies and examples (adopted from HGIP 1994)** (*continued*)	**Primary prevention**	**Secondary prevention**
	A CSE social biology course with the three objectives of education/ information, self-awareness, and counselling.[3]	Some forms of psychotherapy and counselling, particularly those with an educative quality, promoting emotional literacy,[7] emotional education,[8] and somatic education.[9]
	Milton Keynes MIND'S Education Project[4]	
	Campaigns, conferences, booklets, journals, mental health/education weeks/roadshows, seminars, etc.	Counselling in primary care settings
	Mental illness prevention	
	Concerned with targeting vulnerable or 'at risk' groups. *Example:* Mental health at work.	Early detection, management and treatment, including primary care settings. *Example:* Reactive interventions to reduce the risk of developing mental illness

[1]Murray MC (1989) Mental Health Promotion Team. Mid Staffordshire Mental Health Promotion Team.
[2]Kennedy A (1988) *Positive Mental Health Promotion – Fantasy or Reality?* Glasgow: Greater Glasgow Health Board Health Education Department.
[3]Higgins P (1984) Mental health education. *Nursing Mirror*, no. 159: 28–29.
[4]Milton Keynes MIND Education Project, Milton Keynes.
[5]Gatherer A (1963) The Northampton Mental Health Project 1961. An Experiment in Mental Health Education.
[6]Doyle R (1989) A meeting of minds. *The Health Services Journal*, 16, Nov., p.1407.
[7]Steiner C (1984) Emotional literacy. *Transactional Analysis Journal*, **14**: 162–173.
[8]Rakusen J (1990) Emotional education. *Open MIND*, **46**: 10–11.
[9]Keleman S (1989) *Patterns of Distress*. Berkeley, Centre Press.

Nurses and the Health of the Nation

The second Progress Report on the Health of the Nation, *Fit for the Future* (DOH 1995d), applauds the success of the national health strategy and states that 'Effective communication of health messages is about giving people information they need to make their own health choices.' However, choice is only feasible if the foundations for health are in place (see Chapter 1). Furthermore, the relevance of mental health prevention and education does not lie solely at the door of mental health nursing as a specialism. On the contrary, a brief look at the key areas reveals a mental health thread running through them all. Health of the Nation highlights five areas for promoting health and it can be seen that these key areas all have a mental health component (Box 6.3).

Box 6.3

Key area	Mental health link
Coronary heart disease and stroke	Stress
Cancers	Stress/loss
Mental illness	MHP
HIV/AIDS and sexual health	Self-esteem
Accidents	Loss

The state perspective, in terms of education, is one of enabling people to make choices about healthy lifestyle through formal health education programmes and contacts with patients and clients. The contribution of nurses, health visitors and midwives (DOH 1994b) is described as being able to improve recognition, management and treatment of mental illness. With the contribution to changing behaviour, the focus is on 'improving the public understanding of mental illness' and, 'changing the behaviour of the general public, particularly about managing stress'. The contribution to changing practice is seen at several levels:

- Responsiveness to the individual needs of the mentally ill and awareness of signs of risk of suicide
- Improving the continuity of patient care, through greater collaboration with other professions and agencies
- Providing greater levels of support for patients, relatives/carers and health care professionals

What, then, could educative and preventive approaches to mental health look like for nursing as a professional group? Some suggestions are provided in Table 6.5, taking into account the location and specialism of different aspects of the profession.

Table 6.5
MHP for nursing

Area of nursing	Recommendation/focus
District nursing	Clinical audit, guidelines and protocols for practice *Action:* audit of current activity and identification of gaps
General practice	Population approaches to primary prevention and a social context of health
Health visitors	Health promotion/prevention activity; specified and research outcomes of work in areas of poverty/nonpoverty

(*continued overleaf*)

	Area of nursing	Recommendation/focus
Table 6.5 **MHP for nursing** (*continued*)	Learning disability/mental health nursing	Community participation – involvement of local communities in planning of services. *Action:* Inpatient and residential – establish and support community forums and advocacy
	Midwifery nursing	Primary preventive education, client participation and needs assessment
	Occupational health nursing	Men's health and workplace policy development Workplace mental health policy Stress and mental well-being of employees (see *Mental Health at Work, Health of the Nation at Work*, DOH 1996b)
	School nursing	Assessing effectiveness of interventions and adoption of a population approach
	Secondary care nursing	Hospital-based health promotion and enhancing dialogue with primary care Looking at issues of poverty and discrimination
	Specialist nursing	Vehicle to link a health-promoting hospital with community-orientated primary care

In order to examine practically some of the strengths and weakness in a preventive/educational approach to mental health, the example of a national initiative needs to be considered. The national Defeat Depression Campaign will be discussed. This is a public education campaign developed by professional staff.

Depression and MHP: a preventive–educative approach

Context

The rationale for protocols and guidelines around the detection, treatment and management of depression find their roots in government policy and professional services' responses to those policies in the form of a primary care focus and the need to meet the prevention targets set out by the national health strategy. Guidelines are seen in terms of the application of evidence-based medicine and reduction in clinical variability resulting in better patient care.

The UK programme

The British Association of Psychopharmacology (1993) highlights that depression is a common illness affecting 3% of the population per year, and 25% of those with depression do not consult their GP. While acknowledging that environmental and life events factors can precipitate or exacerbate depression, it recommends antidepressant treatment for all depression for at least 4 months. A recent publication by the Nuffield Institute (1993) provides a review of literature on depression and its treatment. It acknowledges that depressive episodes are strongly associated with adverse social and economic circumstances including unemployment, divorce and separation, inadequate housing and lower social class.

Recommendations include establishing clinical guidelines, and the report proposes that a range of statutory agencies should 'identify ways in which coordinated interventions in the health and social spheres can be developed to help depressed individuals, and populations with high rates of depression' (p.7).

The campaign

The Defeat Depression Campaign was begun in 1992 by the Royal College of Psychiatrists in association with the Royal College of General Practitioners. Consensus statements on the treatment of depression in primary care were published in 1995 by the colleges. The campaign has three objectives:

- To increase the knowledge of GPs and other health care professionals in the recognition and effective treatment of depressive illness
- To enhance public awareness of the nature, course and treatment of depressive disorders
- To reduce the stigma associated with depression

Thus, it is aimed at professional health care staff – specialist and otherwise – and the general public. Baldwin and Priest (1995) provide a review of the national campaign, giving background to the initiative, its objectives and possible future activity. Their report examines the evaluation of the campaign and the future direction of such activity. It confesses that measures of evaluation are problematic.

Discussion

One area the campaign has failed to explore is community and individual concerns in relation to the consensus statements. The campaign favour the treatment of depression with appropriate doses of antidepressant medication. The reality is that these are psychoactive drugs and it is imperative that, despite their apparent reliability and safety, a fully informed choice should be arrived at between the recipient and the prescriber. There is also the problem that the prescribing policy of the campaign may allow a primary health care-led NHS and the wider primary health care team to see psychoactive medication as the panacea to emotional ills. Whatever the effect of such drugs on sleeping patterns and mood, they will not alleviate poverty, discrimination and inequality. If they are to be prescribed at all, it is essential that it is to a person who will benefit, who is offered choices. The 'treatment' may go beyond the skills or scope of the primary health care team, but they are in an invaluable position to highlight and direct the person to other forms of assistance, both emotional and practical.

Green (1992) raises concerns about depression becoming commodified with an image problem that can be solved by a new brand name. This brings us back to some of the concerns expressed about poor-quality public health programmes, such as victim-blaming approaches, reinforcement of fatalism, a sense of despair and a one-dimensional response to multiple health needs.

In conclusion it is recognized for the future of the campaign that similar educational strategies such as the 'Gotland effect', although effective, require sustained educational programmes to be most effective.

Other options

A Fellowship has been established to raise the profile of depression for practitioners. A regional network of RCGP Fellows is to be developed and support given to primary health care facilitators. As Baldwin and Priest (1995) state;

> Self-help groups may come to have a special role in complementing the activities of any future educational initiative. Although pharmacological treatments and certain psychological therapies have proven value in the treatment of depression, much of the need of depressed patients remains unmet. (p.75)

Another way forward might be to learn from an initiative around depression in Ireland in 1985 which began via the establishment of a voluntary organization called 'Aware'. The emphasis in the Irish experience is more active involvement of patients and families as well as health professionals. And as early as 1989 the Good Practices in Mental Health Organization published criteria for good quality mental health services in a primary care setting which included user consultation and participation in decision making.

There remain issues in terms of true alliances between the statutory and the voluntary sector in relation to depression. There is the problem that a focus on clinical depression can exclude voluntary agencies and community approaches that may alleviate, explore or analyse the roots of depression and so remove it from political and other action. In short, we can focus on a medical condition and fail to take full account of the social underpinnings of depression and the meaning of depression in society. The inherent tension caused by giving too much emphasis to policy and strategy, at government level, results in a complex mix of outcomes. There is a need to redirect and focus the attention, particularly of specialist mental health services, towards interventions with people experiencing severe mental ill-health and, at the same time, broaden the parameters of nonspecialists and other agencies to pick up the rest of the wider mental health needs of the population. Mental illness service provision has to be considered as part of a strategic approach to mental health. Since psychiatry will continue to have an integral role to play, it is prudent not to exclude its professional expertise. The value of research and evaluation in this field is a prerequisite both for the care of those who are experiencing mental illness and for the development of partnerships at all levels of involvement.

Conclusion

Tudor's (1996) analysis of mental health promotion and the difference between it and community mental health and mental illness casts light on the use of terminology and practice. One of the difficulties for health promotion has been the assumption that prevention is synonymous with promoting health. This excludes the concept of positive health and well-being. While this concept may have its critics, it does demonstrate the importance of clarity in the terminology, the model, the philosophy and the ultimate practice delivered in the field.

A preventive and educative approach to mental illness may prove effective (if only for the practitioners' peace of mind), but what are the long-term consequences of turning our backs on the socio-economic and political roots of mental distress and mental disorder? If we do not address issues of poverty and discrimination we not only condemn the presently exposed to further difficulties but we also fail to consider the impact upon other generations. In the next chapter we examine another key area for influence – the purchasing agenda for health.

Practice checklist

The potential MHP worker can do the following in the area of prevention and education:

- Understand the strengths and weaknesses of the approach

- Recognize that there are no quick fix solutions to mental distress and mental illness

- Be critical of state policy with its emphasis on prevention from a medical perspective, but recognize that the policy focus of primary care (at the secondary level) has implications for innovation within the primary and secondary care interface

Prevention and education often mean information. Identify innovative and participatory methods of sharing information on positive mental health.

Audit activity that is focused at the preventive and/or educative elements. What constitutes your practice? How is it informed?

What elements of your practice do you consider include prevention and preventive methods?

Is there a right balance in your practice between those who are already ill and those whom you may be able to influence?

Can you identify any preventive practice in your area?

What resources, skills and opportunities would you require to develop a preventive approach?

Can education on its own be seen as a preventive intervention?

What do you think are the problems with prevention?

Consider the use of preventive service and approaches more likely to be taken up by an 'articulate' individual or community.

Social isolation is considered as one of the problems most difficult to address and ameliorate as we move into the twenty-first century. It is difficult to see how community responsibility for individuals can have any real worth while the infrastructure is so fragile and rife with inequality. Consider the impact of social isolation throughout the life cycle.

Think about the resources you know in your area for each grouping, however you define them.

How could you compile a directory of relevant workers and organizations to support vulnerable and isolated individuals and groups which could more positively support your role as health promoter? (For example, do you have a black advocacy worker to whom you could refer your clients, or are you aware of a black mental health agency in your area of working practice ?

Would you be prepared to compile a directory of relevant workers and organizations? If not consider whether this is due to the enormity of the task, your lack of skills in this area, lack of education about mental health promotion on your course of training, or an overemphasis on mental illness in enhancing professional competence.

7 Purchasing and MHP

There certainly needs to be a creative tension and robust negotiation between purchasers and providers. But market relationships in the private sector are also built on partnerships and long-term agreements. (Dr Brian Mawhinney, Secretary of State for Health in NHSME, 1993)

Key themes:
- What is health purchasing and who does it involve?
- Purchasing and MHP – the significance
- Examples from practice

Overview

This chapter demonstrates how purchaser and provider arrangements, established as part of NHS reforms of the 1980s, can benefit the mental health of whole populations and specific groups and communities. It consists of a resumé of the purchaser and provider relationship and the respective roles and opportunities for influencing decision-making processes. The context includes government perspectives on purchasing and examples from Trent and South West Region for Mental Health promotion. The chapter will enable a clearer distinction between purchasing and providing to be made and the possible intervention points for influence and critique of the system as it stands. A range of considerations and cues for the purchasing agenda will be made for the health professional and the nonspecialist and community perspectives.

Purchasing and commissioning for health

The reforms of the 1980s have resulted in a separation of managerial roles into purchasing – more recently referred to as commissioning – and the provision of health care. A health purchaser is an agency that is responsible for buying health services to meet the needs of their local population. A health provider is an agency responsible for directly providing services which they 'sell' to purchasers (Medical Campaign Project 1990). Purchasing has been both a response to and an effect of the NHS reforms of the 1980s, culminating in the White Paper *Working for Patients* (DOH 1989b). This divided the functions of health authorities (purchasers) and NHS service provision (trusts as providers). This new set of relations can be set out as in Table 7.1.

Purchaser	Provider	Service receiver
Health authority/ fundholding GP	Trust or a voluntary/ independent agency	General public as actual or potential clients/patients
Assesses local health needs and sets a contract to meet those needs	Agrees a contract and fulfils it by providing a service	

Table 7.1
Provider/purchaser relationships

The purchasing of health care involves three key parties:

- Health authorities
- Trusts and GP fundholders
- Other agencies (independent and charitable) which provide services and the public themselves

The key element is the contract and the contractual obligation between all three parties, although in reality this is more usually between the health authority and the provider. Services are contracted and delivered *on behalf of* individuals, groups and communities. In this sense, despite the apparent marketplace economics of the system, the purchasers and providers, on the whole, remain public services, managed and provided by public servants. However, purchasing is more than making contracts for certain services. The intention of such a model is also that of improving both the access and quality of the services. This is achieved by outcome-based health service provision and broadening of the interpretation of what constitutes services, thereby allowing the independent, private and voluntary sectors into mainstream provision. This should result in a mixed economy of care complete with competition for contracts, although it is assumed that the bulk of services will continue to be provided by the NHS.

This new scenario has implications for all parties concerned:

- The health authority has a new relationship with the providers of services – a contractual one which aims to improve the cost-effectiveness, delivery and quality of health service provision.

- Providers have to respond to this new structure in terms of 'winning' contracts and fulfilling them satisfactorily and being monitored in the process.
- The public are being drawn into the process of assessment of health needs through consultation and participation and views on the quality of services.

Purchasing and MHP: the significance

The role of purchasing within the arena of mental health promotion is significant for several reasons:

1. Within the national health strategy are clear statements and references to prevention, education and promotion in the key area of mental illness. Approaches and interventions suggested are informed by the purchaser and provider process
2. The Community Care Act and other legislation at the health policy level have emphasized the need for strategic responses to the planning and implementation of services. This too can be broadened to include, at the least, quality standards issues that are of relevance to MHP and, more widely, to incorporate issues of advocacy and empowerment
3. The implications of the requirement of health authorities to purchase in terms of health needs for what constitutes a good mental health service.

From the perspective of the general public, purchasing can be seen as a tool for delivering diversity and higher-quality services and alternatives to traditional services. The services purchased on their behalf should be based on objective analysis (in this case mental health as well as mental illness needs assessment). This is why the important elements stressed in Chapters 3 and 4 highlight the need to take account of felt needs and views. There may be no 'scientific' basis of racism influencing the esteem and mental health of a population, but it is what local black people will cite and raise as testimony to their distress. For this reason, regardless of its measurability, it becomes a 'health' issue which needs to be considered alongside morbidity data and mental illness prevalence rates.

From the view of professional health and social care workers, purchasing may seem a remote or an intrusive bureaucratic exercise. However, it effects what, where and how practice takes place. Individuals and teams are close to the causes and sources of and solutions to mental distress. As such it is vital that they take the opportunity to influence purchasing at practical and pragmatic levels.

The state is interested in delivering health policy reforms in a way which is palatable and with the minimum disruption. Key to its philosophy is effectiveness in terms of overall efficiency and cost. While the ideal outcome is the smooth application of purchasing as a philosophy and practice, some of the tensions that the new arrangements create are both inevitable and part of a process of cultural and organizational change.

In order to clarify government policy in relation to the new mechanisms, it is useful to remind ourselves of the thinking that took place as part of the reforms and of contemporary views on the roles of health authorities and health promotion. To explain the process of purchasing and possible ways to influence it, we begin with a resumé of key speeches made by Secretary of State for Health Dr B. Mawhinney in 1993.

The Mawhinney speeches: setting out the market stall

The then Secretary of State for Health set out the government view in relation to purchasing through several key speeches. These have laid the foundation for the building of roles and relations as part of the new agenda promised by the NHS reforms. In these speeches, purchasing is described as: 'the engine that would drive the reforms' (Mawhinney in NHSME 1993, p.11). At a speech given to South Western Regional Health Authority, purchasers are seen as having the three goals outlined in Box 7.1.

Box 7.1 **The three goals for purchasers**

1. To improve people's health by targeting resources on effective ways of delivering clinical care and promoting health

2. Purchasing to improve the quality of health care, making it more responsive to the needs and wishes of people

3. Purchasing to ensure that as many people as possible receive high quality care from what available resources can provide.

Mawhinney (in NHSME 1993, p.38)

The purpose of purchasing, then, is seen as to improve health and health services and to modify inappropriate ways of delivering clinical care and preventing illness. Contracts are seen to be essential to engage providers of services in health promotion. Several key elements are demanded of contracting: to achieve improvements in value for money, effectiveness and quality of services. Dr Mawhinney also set out seven elements for effective purchasing (Box 7.2).

Box 7.2 **Seven 'stepping stones' to successful purchasing**

1. **Strategy:** Long-term purchasing intentions, health targets and measurement
2. **Effective contracts:** Quality and value for money
3. **Knowledge base:** Improving information and intelligence, including providers
4. **Responsiveness to local people:** The public and patients having a say and improving the public's awareness of health and health issues
5. **Mature relations with providers:** Purchasing is about managing relationships and not about buying things. This requires practitioners to be involved in the contracting and monitoring process
6. **Local alliances:** Practical joint activity with other agencies and sharing of skills
7. **Occupational capacity:** 'Organizational fitness' of health authorities to make purchasing achieve its objectives.

As part of the new arrangements it is anticipated that a mixed economy will develop, producing limited 'competition' in the health care arena. Again, this is thought both to improve quality and range of services and to be cost-effective. The current Secretary of State for Health, Frank Dobson, has called for a fundamental review of NHS spending over the next four years. This may result in further changes to the purchasing scenario. A shrewd practitioner should inform oneself of the context in which the previous Government developed purchasing and how it is likely to be modified.

Effective purchasing

Hunter and Harrison (1993) define effective health purchasing as: 'the utilization of the purchaser–provider split so as to enhance the effectiveness and cost effectiveness of health care, responsiveness to the public and the efficiency with which resources are utilized' (p.2). They elaborate on this definition to include the influencing of agencies with a degree of influence over variables which impact on health status, or 'health advocacy'. This suggests that health purchasing is more than a reorganization of services to reduce costs. While economic benefits are anticipated, the reforms and restructuring have more to offer. This is important if we are to consider purchasing for mental health and its promotion.

What is health advocacy?

1. A range of interagency liaison arrangements
2. Clear identification of non-NHS activities and agencies impacting on health
3. Getting health on to the agendas of other agencies.

(Hunter and Harrison 1993)

Ranade (1994) details the willingness of the new system to draw upon the language, ideology and practice of commercial approaches to health care. The apparent transfer is not without cost. The range of terms in use – such as 'patient', 'consumer', 'customer' or 'client' – suggests that different models are in operation. Ranade remains doubtful about the impact on quality of service provision the reforms have had. For instance, what do we mean by 'quality' in the context of psychiatric care in a hospital, of care in a community setting, or of care by a GP?

Critical stance

Ranade (1994) reminds us that the language of health purchasing – value for money, quality, contracts – is framed in a particular view of organizational style and philosophy. Health has become more businesslike to improve the use of the vast quantities of money that it consumes each year. By borrowing both the language and the practice of private, commercial approaches to running and delivering services, significant improvements can be made both practically, culturally and politically. Or so it seems. At its essence are the apparent strengths of cost-effectiveness and robust management which are the hallmarks of successful and competitive businesses. The core of purchasing for the NHS is to emulate such philosophy and practice and ensure that the culture, style and activities of this enormous organization are made more marketlike. The intention was to learn from management theory and practice which placed great emphasis upon target setting, strategy, quality and high-quality management to achieve its ends. The ends in this case are not profits for shareholders but a better-managed and more productive health service delivery and a more meaningfully focused array of services to the population. The creation of trusts and health authorities and general practitioners as purchasers in a contractual relationship with hospital and community service provision was the cornerstone of the government's approach to the NHS. This enabled it to fit within the prevailing ideology of government and also to meet the growing demands on the NHS. One could argue that effective purchasing via a process of sophisticated assessment of need will result in a form of rationing or a moral rationale as where and to whom go finite resources for infinite health issues. Much is expected of purchasing to reshape the historical disciplines and approaches to work for the provider of mental health services. Dr Mawhinney defined effective purchasing in terms of whether it has delivered 'demonstrable improvements' in health. This not only has implications for how we plan ahead for purchasing to ensure that the most effective service is

How do you think the new purchasing arrangements have affected your practice?

What can voluntary and user agencies in mental health hope to benefit from in the NHS from these new arrangements?

purchased but also requires that a range of mechanisms within the private sector, such as quality standards, monitoring and competition, be in place to achieve this in the first place.

Role of the health authority as purchaser

Health authorities provide a strategic overview. They can assess need, make sound projections and determine priorities on the basis of large populations. They also have a vital role-management relationship with the centre. They are the main vehicle – in a publicly financed service – for implementing central priorities such as the Health of the Nation Strategy, the Patients' Charter and Care in the Community. (Mawhinney in NHSME 1993, p.14)

The role of the contemporary health authority according to Hamlin (1996) consists of interagency work, promoting health, determining health policy, assessing health needs, commissioning and monitoring service provision. To achieve this, she argues, the organization needs at once both to be strategic and to adopt a more facilitative style. Let us look at these roles in closer detail, drawing on mental health as an example.

Interagency work

The voluntary and user sector is particularly adept at interagency work, as a necessity and to sustain its activities. Statutory agencies in community and institutional settings have strong histories of multidisciplinary working and team approaches which put them in a favourable position to network with other services and organizations.

Promoting health

Promotion of health occurs by design and by default, especially in the shape of self-help and political lobbying on a range of mental health and health-related issues that individuals and groups embark upon. This valuable experience can enable statutory agencies to view health from a much broader perspective than illness and treatment. Statutory services, on the other hand, have both the personnel and the infrastructure to positively influence the health of the people they come into contact with for mental health treatment and care. Through health alliances they can also influence health from a wider perspective.

Determining health policy

Organizations such as Community Health Councils, MIND, National Schizophrenia Fellowship and SANE highlight policy issues and policy implications at national and local levels. These organizations and the voluntary and user sector can also lobby committees and use the media for exposure of health issues. Statutory agencies are also in a prime position to give practical insights into the opportunities and realities of health policy for the public they serve. Information sharing and genuine dialogue with the user and voluntary sector can make constructive criticism, praise and problem solving for policy implementation a practical reality.

Assessing health needs

The user and voluntary sector together with a range of service providers have considerable local qualitative data on services, service gaps and good practice options. Statutory agencies also have close contacts with individuals and communities which can significantly contribute to the mental health needs assessment process.

Commissioning and monitoring service provision

Via the above processes the voluntary and user sector should be able to influence what services are commissioned, and they are also in an ideal position to report upon service impact. Agencies themselves can engage the user and voluntary services to highlight strengths and weaknesses in mental health service provision.

Purchasing and health promotion

In describing the role of health authorities, Adams (1996) sees the significant policy, operational and organizational changes as having many positive implications for promoting health. She identifies several aims of a health authority: to develop health strategies, to secure services for the public and to engage in public health advocacy. This should be done in a participatory way, requiring the establishment and nurturing of health alliances and interagency partnerships to achieve aims and outcomes (see Chapter 3). For Adams the key features of the new health authority in promoting health rather than managing and commissioning illness and care services requires a political role, one of negotiation and influence which inevitably results in broad social model definition of health and its promotion.

Promotion of mental health from within the structure of a purchasing organization – a health authority – occurs through the purchasing functions of the system, through providers of services and via health alliances. Purchasing of services and influencing of services can focus on population groups, specific health issues, foundations for health and communities as settings and targets for health-promoting activity.

Context to practice

What can the MHP practitioner make of this? In the earlier chapters we have said that it is important to be aware of national and local policy and strategy and to maximize community participation and prevention and education strategies. What purchasing offers is an opportunity for health authorities, the public whom they serve, and service providers to influence the direction of funding and the direction of services. Unlike a health alliance approach, which can be limited to reconfiguring organizational style and the approach to considering and responding to health issues, purchasing actively seeks both to determine health needs and to invest (and disinvest) accordingly. The formulation and monitoring of the contract relationships developed in the system appear to be areas for positive exploitation. This is demonstrated by Mohammed (1993). He acknowledges that purchasing gives an opportunity to examine how improvements in health services for the general population, and more particularly for black communities, can be achieved through the contracting process. At another level, in Anglia and Oxford, Conway *et al.* (1994), as part of a Regional Health development project, state that 'Purchasers should enhance their capabilities and willingness to be "in other people's worlds"' (p.29). This is deemed important in order for them to appreciate the political pressures that are exerted upon themselves and others. This aspect of *being in other worlds* is vital as its extends not just to an appreciation of clinical interventions and operational management of mental illness treatment services. It can potentially go beyond that and extend into the views and experiences of the user, in the voluntary and self-help sector as well as non-NHS services and organizations. This report sets out twelve activities and processes which are seen as essential to good purchasing. In Table 7.2 we have adapted the list to interpret the meaning of effective purchasing for promoting mental health. The examples in italics are opportunities for the agenda or intentions of the purchaser to be influenced for MHP.

Table 7.2
**Aspects of purchasing
and focus for MHP**

(continued opposite)

Activity	Focus
Vision	A clear sense of what the purchaser wants for a population and sharing this with all stakeholders (*User groups carers, housing, GPs, CMHTs*)
Understanding where we are	Information systems, clear objectives and a 'business' sense of health care (*Awareness of policy and other health service changes*)

Activity	Focus	
Strategic scanning	Using epidemiological data and also local and national political developments (*Providers and user movement to do this too, e.g. MIND campaigns on Community Care*)	Table 7.2 **Aspects of purchasing and focus for MHP** (*continued*)
Fundamental rethinking of services	Rethinking provision in its social context e.g. good public health function (*Exploit this role and state the social case*)	
Review	Review the experience with all stakeholders (*An inclusive approach with the user, voluntary sector genuinely involved*)	
Health strategy	Construction of a 3–5 year view of purchaser intentions (*Lobby for involvement in this process*)	
Planning and contracting	Dividing strategy into short-term steps, setting priorities and negotiating with providers (*Identify ways to influence this process*)	
Setting standards	Being clear about how they are to be attained and monitoring their implementation (*What do user surveys, clinical research say regarding this?*)	
Evaluation and monitoring	Comparing data with standards required to 'generate learning' (*This learning to go beyond the confines of a health authority*)	
Influencing	Via collaboration, dialogue, partnerships, advocacy and alliances (*Positively exploit this need of the purchaser*)	
Developing capability	Developing purchaser and network partners (*Request training, support and guidance*)	
Managing continuity and change	Good management systems and creatively dealing with conflict (*This is another area of expertise for good community mental health work*)	

Key themes from this table are the issues of participation and communication: good formal relationships with agencies contracted with and also the wider stakeholder networks. The system – the purchasing market economy that is a result of health and social policy – cannot function without the influence of stakeholders and the wider agenda. This allows a broader definition of health to be considered: everything is in the air and there are apparently limitless opportunities to shape and influence purchasing plans and the process of purchasing to take on board issues that are key to promoting mental health.

What, then, are the key elements of purchasing and how can these be influenced?

Key elements of purchasing

Health needs assessment: the role of the purchaser

One of the core tasks of a health authority is to assess the health needs of the public and to purchase services according to those needs. This can be as innovative or as narrow as one wishes. As discussed in Chapters 3 and 4, 'felt needs' are important and the participation of community and community of interest in the formulation of needs assessment exercises is desirable. Explicit references in a range of policy and supporting documentation from the government and other departments stress the importance of such participation and involvement in a range of planning and decision making processes. The range includes economic plans as part of the national Single Regeneration Budget (SRB) scheme with tenancy and community involvement; strategies such as Tackling Drugs Together which refer to the importance of interagency and community dialogue; and specific mental health and health-related policy and strategy such as Community Care and the Mental Illness Key Area together with local purchasing intentions.

The Leeds Declaration

The Leeds Declaration (1994) raises the issue of how to undertake such an approach considering the qualitative as well as the epidemiological, scientific measurement of health needs. Given the subjective element of health *per se* and of emotional health and well-being and the factors which can inhibit or promote it, this seems a relevant approach to take (see Box 7.3). It also allows for broader definitions of health to be considered and for a social model of mental health to be an inextricable complement of the needs assessment process and purchasing intentions.

Box 7.3 **The Leeds Declaration. New ways to understand and solve public health problems**

> The declaration poses four questions to highlight the significance of a range of methods to understand and manage public health.
>
> *What information do we want?*
> Evidence points to economic, social and political factors being the basis of ill-health and disease. This also requires investigation of why some people remain healthy despite not having foundations for health.
>
> *How do we find out what we need to know?*
> Information about health requires traditional methods and subjective testimony. This qualitative approach should be developed into as robust a methodology as standard approaches.
>
> *Who should we work with?*
> The use of lay workers in research should be encouraged, and also of people from health and social sciences.
>
> *What should we do with the information we receive?*
> 'Research of itself will do nothing to change people's lives and it is important to ensure that all the discoveries about the causes of ill-health are utilized to promote better health.'

Thus, needs assessment can include community participation and community development approaches to assessing health needs and also includes more top-down initiatives which have come in the wake of the reforms such as the Patients' Charter and Local Voices. Methods can range from surveys of users and the local catchment population, the use of focus groups and interviews, as well as, for example, GP referral patterns. Opportunities for influencing the mental health promotion agenda are considerable.

From a traditional mental illness service perspective, Conway *et al.* (1994) have usefully produced a one-year prevalence of psychiatric morbidity in an average purchasing authority with a population of half a million. This highlights the significant role that primary care can and will contribute in this area. The authors point out that twice the average prevalence will occur in economically deprived areas. One issue raised again, as it is by other nursing and purchasing authors, is the importance for mental health staff, especially CPNs and related practitioners, to focus their skills on the people most at need – that is people with acute and enduring mental illness. We would argue that it is this focus that allows opportunities to promote the mental and emotional well-being of people with established mental ill-health. These are core health service care provision issues, but given the public health advocacy role and influence as set out by the Anglian report (Conway *et al.* 1994), it is clear that purchasing goes beyond a reductionist approach to illness and the reproduction of traditional modes of delivery.

Health needs assessment is also required to establish purchasing intentions and plans in order to meet government policy. The action summary in Chapter 3 of the Key Area Handbook: Mental Illness (DOH 1993a) stipulates the importance of developing a local population profile to build up what it terms a 'composite picture' of mental health needs to meet Health of the Nation targets. It proposes establishing a population profile, assessing the needs of people with mental illness and identifying initiatives and service available. It suggests this should be done in collaboration with GP fundholders to improve awareness from a primary as well as a specialist perspective. Six areas for population profile are proposed, matching Health of the Nation targets:

1. Areas of high unemployment, with a focus on young men
2. Alcohol consumption and substance misuse
3. The proportion and location of people from black and other ethnic minorities, including refugees, and whether they are established in or new to the United Kingdom
4. Areas of poor housing, overcrowding and lack of amenities
5. Numbers of people who are elderly and very elderly
6. Numbers of single parents and children in single-parent families.

The Key Area Handbook stresses that the needs assessment processes should be 'sensitive' to differences of age, gender, social class and ethnicity as well as to general care needs associated with specific mental illness. Table 7.3 adapted from the Key Area Handbook considers needs assessment taking into account particular sensitivities of groups.

Table 7.3
Issues to be considered when assessing needs of particular population groups and communities (adapted from DOH 1993a)

Group	Issue
People from black and other ethnic minorities	Professionals from similar cultural backgrounds Interpreting services Culturally specific requirements
Women	Access to child care facilities at day centres or outpatient clinics, etc. The choice of a female professional, including a female keyworker The choice of a single-sex ward (or area within a ward)
Mentally disordered offenders	Local and medium-secure hospital provision at all levels Nonsecure provision

(continued opposite)

Group	Issue
Older adults	Practical advice and support for carers Continuing and terminal care beds for people with dementia Respite care
Children and adolescents	The rate and effect of changes in family circumstance such as separation, divorce or death of a parent The level of homelessness and poor living conditions Substance misuse in children/adolescents and their parents
Other groups	People who are homeless Carers of people with mental illness People with both physical and mental illness People with learning disabilities and mental illness Lesbians and gay men

Table 7.3
Issues to be considered when assessing needs of particular population groups and communities (adapted from DOH 1993a)
(continued)

The importance of sensitivity to particular groups' needs should not be underestimated, nor should historical and organizational responses to those needs be downplayed. The process of a needs assessment exercise, as with community development and community participation, requires tact and empathy to ensure that such an undertaking does not result in simplistic reproduction of racial, sexual or ageist stereotypes. The 'health' needs of populations can tell us as much about the effectiveness, or otherwise, of service provision as can the 'illness' needs of individuals. The development of a local health needs profile can assist statutory agencies (including purchasers) to identify sources of help and initiatives aimed at promoting the mental health of the local population. According to the Key Area this can include the following:

- Health education across age groups in formal and informal settings
- Media coverage of mental health issues
- Training opportunities for professionals and lay people, such as teachers, carers, youth workers
- Information on mental health and mental illness available to the general public and service users
- Job creation schemes and activities for the unemployed
- Support projects for single parents
- Local suicide support services
- Community and leisure facilities

Health needs assessment tends to be illness-oriented rather than health-focused. How would you look at the mental health needs of a given population or locality? What would you consider and what process would you go through in order to identify local need?

The list is potentially endless and reinforces the importance of taking both a holistic and a health alliance approach to mental illness prevention and the promotion of mental health. Health needs assessment is in many respects the foundation for effective purchasing of health and illness services. It is also an exercise that needs to be repeated and refined as groups and populations fluctuate and as the environments they live in alter or are affected by, for example, employment changes, housing redevelopment or other factors. Assessment of health needs, then, feeds into the contracting process which we will now briefly describe.

The contracting process

There are a range of models outlining the commissioning and contracting process: Sang (1994), Malby (1995) on Nursing and Audit, the Health Advisory Service review on Child and Adolescent Mental Health Services (DOH 1995a) and the Faculty of Public Health Medicine report (1996). The last document is particularly relevant in that it spells out the differences between commissioning, purchasing and contracting. Purchasing is seen as the technical procedure used to secure and monitor services from providers. Contracting is defined as a subdivision of this and is the process by which services are purchased from providers. Commissioning has a focus on strategy and includes purchasing and contracting. In this sense it is a 'strategically driven process' (p.71). As we have discussed in previous chapters, this makes the influencing of strategy as well as purchasing an important task in enabling positive action on MHP.

Following our discussion on purchasing and possible intervention points by the public, professionals and users alike, in the next section we examine some examples of good practice which demonstrate the relevance of purchasing to MHP.

Do you see the purchaser/provider arrangements as improving opportunities for health or as ways of rationing tight health budgets. What is your evidence?

How would you improve value for money, effectiveness and quality of services?

Examples of good practice

User empowerment and purchasing

The area of user participation and influence will be discussed in greater detail in Chapter 8. However, a central theme of purchasing involves, to varying degrees, listening and responding to the voice of actual, potential and previous users of services that are purchased. Not only is their involvement welcomed, the positive consequences of such an approach can themselves be mental health promoting.

A good example of a set of guidelines which can be adapted by both purchasers and service providers alike is that set out in Trent RHA's aid to contracting (NHS Executive Trent 1994a). This examines purchasing from the perspective of user empowerment, which it defines as supporting individual users of mental health services:

> Purchasers of mental health care services need to include effective user empowerment mechanisms in their criteria for contracting, and to work with providers to set and monitor standards of practice. Both must involve representative users and potential users in developing user empowerment appropriate to local population needs. (p.7)

The guide raises possible concern over how lifestyles are perceived by professionals and by decision makers allocating resources. Support and training are recommended to deal with this potential discrimination. It also suggests consciousness of risk indicators and vulnerable groups in relation to user empowerment: social factors, women, age, black and ethnic minorities, homeless people, and children and adolescents. In terms of contracting, the guide sees the purchasing role as developing service specification in consultation with users, including their involvement in monitoring mechanisms.

The Trent Regional MHP Group

An example of mental health promotion and purchasing is focused in the work of a regional group consisting of health promotion specialists, psychology, and nurse managers/practitioners at Trent. The categories developed by the Regional MHP Group as part of an attempt to audit activity are outlined in Box 7.4.

Box 7.4 **Trent's MHP audit**

1. Promoting the mental well-being of the general population
2. Preventing mental health problems in vulnerable groups
3. Promoting the well-being of people with mental health problems
4. Promoting the mental well-being of those who have had mental health problems
5. Individuals, groups, agencies and materials concerned with improving the provision for the prevention of mental illness and well-being of the population with mental health problems.

In practice this meant:

- A community mental health roadshow – exhibitions, information and advice
- Involvement of Relate, anxiety management groups, education packages for families, carers and sufferers where schizophrenia has been diagnosed
- Drop-in centres, postnatal support, Community Care projects
- Supported accommodation projects, confidence building groups linking adult education and mental health services
- MHP forums, Community Health Council working parties

Such an auditing process is necessary, particularly when we refer back to the importance of establishing and maintaining health alliances, of intersectoral collaboration and of developing mental health promotion strategy at the broad and specific levels. From the audit of practice, a purchasing document has been developed. This identifies a range of items of service that can contribute to the mental health and well-being of the whole population and specific groups within it. As Magowan states (1994) the purchasing 'shopping list' seeks to highlight key purchasing elements which can be developed into a comprehensive package to promote the mental health of a population. It suggests eight elements which should be present in all NHS contracts:

1. The Patients' Charter
2. An equal opportunities policy
3. Working in partnership with users to develop services
4. Encouraging the development of life-skills and self-efficacy
5. Ensuring access to services by providing information about their availability and promoting what they offer
6. Supporting the personal and professional development of staff and patients
7. Provision of effective communication systems within and between organizations
8. Provision of health promotion activities based on appropriate health needs assessment.

Aside from the eight elements above, the potential 'shopping list' highlights three areas for purchasing (Box 7.5).

Box 7.5 **MHP in Trent – Audit themes and practice**

- Promoting the mental health of the general population: The Public are the key element

- Promoting the mental health of people in vulnerable groups: The key lead agents are the public with the voluntary sector working in combination with professionals and service users
- Promoting the mental health of people in contact with mental illness/psychiatric services: The lead is professionals and mental health specialists but must include the public as carers and recipients and supporters of community care, service users and the voluntary agencies

A range of services – health, social services and others – have been identified as relevant for purchasing MHP under the three elements above:

- Primary health care – general practice services
- Primary health care – community health services
- Mental health services
- Learning disability services
- Acute services
- Health alliances:
     Social services
     Educational services
        (schools, colleges, community education)
     Employers and trades unions
     Voluntary and self-help services

Other elements could be included to reflect local priorities, such as rural versus urban environments. An example is provided to reflect elements for purchasing for primary care (Table 7.4). These three elements of

Table 7.4
Purchasing MHP in primary care for the general population, vulnerable groups and the mentally ill

Promoting the mental health of the general population	Promoting the mental health of people in 'vulnerable groups'	Promoting the mental health of people in contact with mental illness/psychiatric services
Generic counselling services	Specialist counselling services	Training for GPs, prescribing and clinical guidelines
Relief staff to enable primary health care team to attend training	Training of staff in emotional literacy	Updating GPs in mental health treatment and care
Training for staff in communication skills	Training for staff to access welfare rights and advice services	Access by patients to full information on medication and therapies
Training for staff in MHP	Training for stress management	Involvement of users in development of training programmes for staff

MHP can in turn reflect the priorities within the local broad health strategy for Sheffield, Framework for Action (see Chapter 2), which identified 'mental and emotional well-being' as a key area for action.

MHP and purchasing: the South Thames experience

The result of a conference to provide a framework for purchasing MHP was a checklist for purchasers similar to the Trent guideline documents, the menu by the Regional MHP group and the audit of MHP activities discussed earlier. In terms of the South Thames document (Deacon and Dark 1994) the checklist is intended to 'assist the development of a specification for MHP based on understanding and quality of communication.' (p.1)

The checklist identifies six possible outcomes:

1. The long-term outcome of changes in perception and attitudes in the media, young people and the general public
2. Involvement of users in the development of service specification
3. A specification reflecting user needs
4. Information that is appropriate and culturally sensitive
5. Methods of reviewing and evaluating information
6. MHP programmes and campaigns implemented and evaluated.

The checklist is intended to be used by a multiagency groups of purchasers, providers and users and covers a range of themes for MHP. The specification itself asks a range of questions on four areas and asks for an organizational lead and time scale. These areas are:

- Clarifying values for MHP
- Establishing needs and wants
- Developing a specification for MHP
- Setting standards and priorities for MHP

Discrete population groups

Women

There are also documents that identify issues relevant to mental health and its promotion for specific population groups. This is particularly true of the work by Williams *et al.* (1993), who have produced a framework for purchasing effective mental health services for women. This highlights the importance of developing purchasing strategies and contracting with services which are safe, acknowledge 'hidden causes' of distress, promote nondrug treatments and are accessible and community-based. To achieve this, thorough consultation and participation with women as part of the assessment of need, training and contract monitoring are proposed. While the focus is on mental health service provision, issues of quality, access and shaping of services to respond to user needs are paramount. This suggests that the purchasing function can change service provision to make it more appropriate to women's mental health as well as their illness needs.

Purchasing health services for men

The East Midlands Men's Health Network have developed a document (NHS Executive, Trent 1994b) produced by Working with Men, following a National Men's health conference in 1994. This short report suggests that purchasers should consider identifying need and an awareness of research findings on men's health as well as work-based clinics and the implications of class, race, employment status and activity as well as marital status. The final point is the importance of monitoring progress in order to evaluate the effectiveness of clinic-based approaches to reaching men's health needs.

Black mental health and purchasing

Cochrane and Sashidharan (1996), in a review of the literature relating to mental health and ethnic minorities, provide implications for services. They looked at the prevalence rate of schizophrenia in the African-Caribbean population, in-patient admissions of other diagnoses and the low-treated prevalence rates of the South Asian population. Calls are made for improvements in thoroughness of research and in acceptability of services (statutory and voluntary) to the black community. They cite Moodley (1993), who defines an 'ideal service' as one which people trust, which has a racial and cultural mix of staff at all grades, one with availability of interpreters, one whose assessments are not 'Euro centric', and one which provides appropriate information and draws on the strengths and experience of communities. This appears a useful framework in which purchasers can specify what they want from mental health services to meet the needs of ethnic minority communities.

SNMAC primary care public health nursing and purchasing

As the focus of health care shifts towards the primary care sector it is essential for service relationships between the secondary, occupational, private health and social care sectors to be redefined. The public health

> perspective in health promotion and disease and disability prevention, are important linkages to be maintained across sector boundaries. Individually and collectively in teams, the full potential for the nursing contribution to public health should come from interagency, intersectoral, multidisciplinary and community involvement with the primary health sector in centre position.

The creation of the purchaser/provider split for primary care has resulted in the development of the GP fundholding scheme. It is not for this text to discuss the context of this development, but for a thorough review of the issues see Duggan (1995) and North (1995). However, what has been experienced as part of the fundholding development has been the creation of GPs as partial and, in newer experiments, total purchasers able to roam in relative freedom to purchase services for their practice populations. This has implications in terms of influencing these new purchasers. With primary care the focus will be on a smaller locality – the practice population as opposed to large-scale purchasing for population groups such as women's mental health or children's services for a District. The same principles of influence apply, however, and the emphases on quality and patient participation and community development approaches to health ensure that such developments can be informed by an MHP agenda.

Professional staff have a key role in facilitating such a process and can act as a link between purchasing strategy, implementation and activity for the public and users alike. The RCN (1993) in *The Role of Nurses in Purchasing for Health Gain*, highlights that nurses possess skills relevant to the purchasing processes as they can key into the needs assessment process via their direct contacts with communities. As discussed in the section in Chapter 2 on Nursing and Public Health Issues, the document by SNMAC, *Making It Happen* (DOH 1995b) provides thirteen recommendations, nine of which relate to purchasing with a recommendation referring specifically to health promotion: 'Address health promotion in hospital service specifications, and ensure by contract that secondary care providers are systematically incorporating health promotion interventions where there is known health benefit' (Recommendation 8). This suggests that purchasing is the lever to press for change in the culture and practices of staff who deliver services so that they operate in a way that takes direct account of health-promoting activity.

There are dilemmas in this approach. The most obvious is that we fall back upon a limited health promotion and indeed a mental health promotion that is either an improved version of giving information to patients or a narrow adjustment of lifestyle which can compensate for and protect against the stresses of life. SNMAC sees public health in nursing, midwifery and health visiting practice as about commissioning health services and providing professional care and it cites health visiting skills being founded on four principles of practice that have been adapted by the UKCC as the basis for post-registered education. Table 7.5 shows what this could look like for mental health and its promotion and shows the possible contribution that this group of professionals could make.

Health visiting practice	Mental health promoting focus	
1. The search for health needs	Identification of mental health *as well as* illness needs – the search for community strengths and weaknesses in collaboration with local people *as well as* professionals	Table 7.5 **Four principles of practice for health visiting**
2. Stimulating awareness of health needs	Working with local people, agencies and services, coordinating information on mental health, raising mental health issues as *a shared concern*	
3. Encouraging health-enhancing activities	In *partnership* with communities, developing small-scale solutions: group support, befriending	
4. Influencing policies affecting health	In *partnership* with communities, influencing policies affecting mental health	

Two recommendations are made in respect of health visiting. The first is that purchasers of health visitor services should as part of the service specifications include promotional and preventive activity, including information for monitoring health outcomes. The second emphasizes the importance of research into the outcomes of health visitors' work with children and families living in disadvantaged and nondisadvantaged communities. Purchasers of learning disability and mental health nursing are also urged to use contracts to influence requirements for client and carers' participation in operational planning of service provision and delivery.

Conclusion

Our review of the background and process of purchasing reveals a range of intervention points for informing its operation. The climate and the enthusiasm surrounding the reforms and their very process of implementation have resulted in radical shifts and changes in the way in which the NHS is organized and services are provided. However, for the people who use or potentially may use the service, it is very much 'business as usual'. People still have GPs, there are referrals, specialties, clinics and hospitals. And there are also people who do not have access to services, such as the homeless and the vulnerable. The recent changes can appear as little more than cosmetic adaptations to waiting-room environments and limited choices in service. Yet, beneath the surface the changes and the potential for influence are considerable. Despite the references to learning and responding to the needs of service users and the public, this area remains relatively untapped. It is the role of the user and voluntary sector, together with their professional allies, to identify how the reforms can be influenced in order to meet mental health as well as mental illness needs. It is this area of user involvement and power that will be discussed further in the next chapter.

Practice checklist

- Find out what the contracts are for the service you provide: how broad or specific are they? Is there a health promotion requirement? What is the local Community Health Council's view on purchasing strategies for mental health?

- Keep track of local projects and initiatives that are purchaser-led or in collaboration with your agency.

- Is the population you serve aware of what the contract for a service means? Are its members aware of how they could be enabled to inform its development or content?

- Look at ways of identifying mental health as well as mental illness need. What constitutes a mentally healthy community? What would you define as a mentally healthy place to live?

- Remember that your networks, contacts and exposure to local issues are vital intelligence and information. Use this valuable data to inform the purchasing process.

The user focus

8

Health For All is concerned with creating structures and mechanisms that empower and support individuals in developing and using their own capabilities to the fullest extent possible. It aims to enable them to realize their full potential for health and thereby enhance the quality of their lives. (WHO 1991)

Key themes:

- The user movement
- MHP and users
- Self-help – the professional perspective
- The state perspective – seeking local views
- Good practice

Overview

This chapter aims to clarify the health promoter's role, limitations and responsibility in the context of the user movement. It also provides a checklist for good practice and guidelines for involvement in projects and initiatives by a synthesis of the various policy statements of the statutory and voluntary agencies and good practice positions of the user movement and its allies. We explore the potential of initiatives such as the Mental Health Charter developed by the Mental Health Task Force and provide a brief historical overview and policy examination in terms of the relationship between the consumer or user role as outlined in Community Care and the NHS reforms. The primary focus will be initiatives which relate to clear policy guidelines, but the main emphasis is on ordinary citizens, their role in and their ability to participate in and affect change for those suffering the consequences of mental health provision, and on the impossibility of equitable roles in this. The matter of professional involvement of staff in this sensitive area will be debated and solutions to the professional and personal divide will be clarified and solutions proposed.

Introduction

The importance of the user movement and the relevance of user power have a considerable history. A recent survey of 119 trusts in England by the Institute of Health Service Management (Danneman and Howland 1996) examined the extent of user involvement in the 'strategic direction' of health service providers and the extent to which trusts had become 'user friendly'. A minority have mental health users on the board, a third have regular meetings with user representatives. The changes in health policy (see Chapter 2) impacting on how health services are planned and delivered have service users – actual or potential – as key to their vision statements if not their action. The policy push and reforms of the NHS in a climate of 'consumerism' as discussed in the previous chapter, including a consumerism of health and lifestyle, have resulted in the issue of user-defined service provision receiving a prominence unheard of in previous decades. There are also encouraging moves of practical financial assistance to user groups and support for advocacy, and some examples of trusts employing workers to improve user involvement. This issue of practical, financial support is a recurring theme in other studies and reviews. Other types of support are also required. For example, Ross (1995), in research on how effective user involvement in mental health day services takes place, argues that it requires organizational support and valuing of workers.

The issue of user involvement has been prioritized for our discussion because it is key for all parties in the mental health arena and has been identified by statutory, voluntary and user-led organizations alike. The following is a brief resumé of relevant literature and discussions held with a range of service users and projects.

Table 8.1 shows how Pilgrim (1993) sets out the scenario for mental health users in terms of past perceptions and perspectives versus a

Table 8.1
Past and possible scenarios for mental health users

		Past	**Future**
User views		See themselves as disabled/desire for conventional services	See themselves as citizens/ demand for social change and individual support
Social perspectives	Caring, altruistic, Victorian values	Modern, individualistic, holistic	
Professional views	Part of the system	Struggling to develop autonomy for users	
Political options	Incorporated provision	Tolerance, diversity, 'green' solutions	

possible future. It is hoped that a mental health-promoting philosophy and practice (praxis), underpinned by the principles of Health for All, ensures that this is the direction in which we are heading. It also demonstrates the role that users, cultural and public perceptions, practitioners and policy makers have in taking us towards a more user-focused future. The practitioner is a key element in this struggle for autonomy.

The user movement

User involvement and community participation can be seen as having their roots in a range of WHO declarations in relation to citizenship and rights for health. This has been interpreted in a variety of ways by a range of health and social policies (see Chapter 2). In the context of the United Kingdom this has resulted in a national health strategy with mental illness as a key component. Within this are calls for involving users and carers and the development of user-led services. At the operational level this has resulted in changes of emphasis and conceptualization of the terminology of users and power. The conceptualization of users is also evident in the work of health professionals in terms of their role as health promoters and of attempting to prevent mental distress in the first instance.

Hoggert and Hambleton (1987) argue that the shift to make public services more 'user-centred' reveals two separate approaches:

1. Consumerism with a focus on the responsiveness of public services – such as waiting times, complaints and service reliability
2. Collective responses which place more importance on democratizing services.

The first is about tinkering, or improving the performance of services. The second goes further, to the structures and processes of services. In the field of mental illness service provision, a move towards democratization has a considerable appeal.

Sedgwick (1983) provides a survey of the user movement during the 1970s and early 1980s and locates it within a political as well as psychiatric struggle. He argues that change and psychiatric reform have always been connected with conditions of political possibility to be promoted or held back by ideologies and social movements. Pilgrim (1993) acknowledges that it has been a Conservative administration that has introduced a user-led ideology through the health service reforms. The Labour Party initially maintained the medical status quo with a traditionalist focus on beds and service provision. Lobbying by user activists throughout the 1980s has resulted in a potential climate for change, and 'a new political ambivalence about professionally defined policies creates an opportunity for more user friendly services' (p.252).

In contrast, Ong (1993) provides a summary of the National Health Service reforms which refers to user participation in service delivery and planning. He argues that while user views and experiences of services have been encouraged through the legislative changes, this has tended to be limited to user involvement around service quality issues. However, despite such limitations, this is seen as significant in changing practice. Balogh and Bond (1995) give an example of involving users in the development of a system of clinical audit, recognizing the strengths of such an approach in informing professional standards. Rogers *et al.* (1993), in an extensive survey of user views, sees the recent interest in 'patient satisfaction' as influenced by the underlying ideology of health care policy. The prevailing ideology emphasizes the need for services to be accountable to patients, but, as Rogers argues: 'As it stands, present policy is rhetorically about consumers but actually it is about the purchasers of services: that is, health authorities. The latter need only incorporate a consumer perspective when, and if, it is expedient' (p.2). This can result in a limited or paternalistic perception of service users. Within a traditional perspective the users of mental health services views are seen as benefiting the system in terms of clinical or quality audit or as a therapeutic interlude in the traditional interventions of psychiatry. Given the state's control over and compliance with the dominant ideologies of medicine and psychiatry, and the consumerist approach to health care, an increasing politicization of the user movement is inevitable. Campaigning and lobbying skills, combined with alliances between other oppressed groups, have fine-tuned the resolve of user activists (Campbell 1995).

Lindow (1996) provides a review of mental health service user action to make information and ideas accessible to service users. She describes how user-controlled alternatives to statutory services are organized across Europe and the United States. She also outlines several levels of user consultation between individual consumers of services, at project- or ward-based level and in service and district-wide forums (Lindow 1991).

Box 8.1 **Contemporary examples of user-led activity**

- A GP Advocacy Service, run by MIND in Camden and providing an independent advocacy service supporting people with mental health problems when they consult a GP
- The Distress Awareness Training Agency in Manchester, which is a user-led cooperative of trainers

- The Newcastle Mental Health Services Consumer Group, which acts as a forum offering a consumer voice for users of mental health services
- The establishment of a Hearing Voices network for people who experience hallucinations
- Crisis Cards and mobilization of support against legislation to strengthen the supervision of treatment under the Mental Health Act

We now consider the user perspective from international, European and more local perspectives before examining issues of encouraging or hindering a user focus for mental health services and MHP.

Lay participation in health

Brochie and Wann (1993) define the 'lay person' as someone who represents the public at large and whose starting point should be the user's or patient's point of view (p.5). Lay participation in health is described as including self-help groups, the public at large and current users of services: 'The lay person is becoming an increasingly important player in health politics as consumerism and consultation become the common language of health management and policy' (p.6).

Box 8.2 **What lay participation offers**

- Personal experience and common sense
- Specialist information and a different perspective
- An understanding of where and how services need developing in the community
- Enabling of communication between service users and health service providers
- Additional care and support

In order to examine the user perspective on mental health, we now examine the thinking at the international, national and more local levels.

A note on carers and caring

Inevitably the issue of user perspectives will also include elements that impinge upon the lives of people who act as 'conscious carers' and those to whom care 'happens'. We acknowledge that rights and opinions of carer and cared for may conflict; however, the emotional, mental health needs of both parties need to be taken into consideration. A key area for the carer in terms of their mental health is the situation of the person having to support in a variety of ways someone with a physical or mental health problem. The Carers (Recognition and Services) Act 1995 now provides formal recognition of the role that informal carers such as families, friends and neighbours play. Carers are now entitled to an assessment of their needs alongside the assessment made for the people they care for.

The World Health Organization view

The Ottawa Charter for Health Promotion (WHO 1986) defines prerequisites for health and identifies areas for health promotion action including the development of community action as well as personal skill development. Both of these can be related to the area of user involvement. It is also in keeping with a user-led philosophy which places psychiatry in a broader context including a social as well as biological examination and explanation. The Health for All targets as set out by WHO (1991) declare that:

> Health for All is concerned with creating structures and mechanisms that empower and support individuals in developing and using their own capabilities to the fullest extent possible. It aims to enable them to realize their full potential for health and thereby enhance the quality of their lives.

WHO accepts that in areas such as primary care, mental health is a neglected component and that it does not always require specialist treatment or management within a hospital setting. WHO also stresses the importance of involving the community at all levels of planning and development (Declaration in Alma-Ata, WHO 1978).

The European view

Glasman (1991) describes the radical combination of clients and ex-clients in the *clientbond* in Holland in 1971. This arose from a group of parents who fought against the sacking of a psychiatrist from a children's adolescent unit. Two years later the focus had switched from parents to users. Patients' Councils developed in the late 1970s, and in 1981 the National Association of Patients' Councils was created. The Dutch government also funded a National Association of Patients' Advocates that has extended to almost all psychiatric hospitals in Holland. Both the councils and the advocate scheme have basic principles that include speaking only for patients, independence of management, accessibility and being informed and informing. The move towards this has to be seen against the major battles in mental health that have been lost and is in some senses part of the pragmatism of the 1980s and 1990s previously discussed. Thus, the energy is directed at the form of mental health care and its institutions rather than at the content of treatment approaches and regimes. Ultimately, how much say can an empowered user have against the scientific, mythic, political and legislative backdrop that is the reality of psychiatry?

The UK perspective

The user perspective in mental health is given significant emphasis in the reforms and in all government documentation relating to mental health. As part of Health of the Nation, the Mental Health Task Force was set up to facilitate a range of initiatives in the mental health field, including the issue of user and carer involvement. Black (1992) provides a thorough overview of material published on the subject between 1985 and 1992. The Key Area Handbook: Mental Illness (DOH 1993a) is a practical guide to assist in developing local strategies for reaching the targets set in the Health of the Nation and contains a chapter on seeking local views. Local consultation is seen as a vital element of the needs assessment process and of informing the service quality agenda. Such consultation is intended to gather intelligence on services in terms of delivery, access, information and appropriateness. Involving service users is recognized as important, requiring practical assistance to facilitate their involvement. Paying expenses, supporting advocates, user-led groups and availability of information in a range of languages and media are all proposed. Supporting advocacy services via commissioning and service specifications, together with access to senior management, is also suggested to maximize involvement.

The Welsh Planning Forum

The *Protocol for Investment in Health Gain, Mental Health* (NHS Directorate 1993) is written by the Welsh Planning Forum to give expert advice on the planning of health services. Despite this worthy aim, it is significant to note that the membership of the Forum does not include expertise from the user or voluntary sectors. The document sets out its aim in relation to participation in the planning process as being 'to ensure people's needs and expectations are considered when services are being planned'. A detailed account of the importance of involving users is given, including recognition that users have limited access to resources. It stresses that users require payment for transport and alternative carers, administrative support and an infrastructure including paid workers and access to advocacy schemes. Management commitment to the process of consultation is regarded as essential.

The mental health charities' view

The Mental Health Foundation's recent inquiry into creating community care (1994) is frank in its approach to resource issues and the inclusion of service users' views. It was written in response to public concerns over cases of self-harm and harm to others by people with severe mental illness. Themes of choice and consultation are part of the report's recommendations. Issues for mental health service providers discussed include the stance that 'People with severe mental illness are entitled to respect and trust, to information, and to consultation and choice in the provision of services' (p.9). In terms of practical ways forward for a responsive community care service it recommends that 'commissioning authorities establish panels of service users to advise on the development and evaluation of services for people with severe mental illness' (p.54). It argues that this needs to be backed up by support, training and the payment of those users taking part. The national charity MIND has produced its Policy 1 (MIND 1994a) in response to the Health of the Nation and sets out the involvement of users in the national targets. It recommends that organizations commission users to develop assessment protocols and measures of service outcome and quality. Mental health purchasers are urged to build into contracts policies to protect people's rights and service providers to monitor the harm their services do to health and social functioning. A second report by MIND, *The Right to Know* (1994b) is in response to research of user views and calls for a radical change in the practice and attitudes of all professionals in mental health. Full information-giving is seen as vital to health and social care provision and planning.

A regional review

The Health Gain Investment Programme (HGIP 1994) provides guidance to the purchasing and service provision functions of services in the Trent Region in England. Using a thorough literature search of good practice on user-led initiatives, the programme is a useful framework providing practical insights into the importance of recognizing and supporting such initiatives. It highlights the points listed in Box 8.3.

Box 8.3 **Users**

- Users should be involved in all stages of planning, running and evaluating services, including policy formulation

- Mental health services should ensure users feel safe to participate, by introducing effective policies governing confidentiality, complaints and victimization. A single user should not be expected to represent all users. Users can represent their own point of view or that of, say, a self-advocacy group
- Translating commitment to user involvement into practice requires resources and specific practical steps, for example, travel, administration costs, space for users to meet, payment for consultancy services

(HGIP 1994)

The HGIP raises key points for involving users in contracting, and involvement in training issues is also suggested. Voluntary organizations' studies of users' views are also reviewed, raising issues such as the need for better staff and patient relations and the right to be properly informed and treated with respect. Professional studies of users' views, specific treatments, gender, race and carers' perspectives are also provided. Another regional document, *Focus on Promoting Health at Work in the NHS* (Trent Regional Health Authority 1994), sets out guidelines for purchasers. In terms of promoting staff health and the role of voluntary and self-help organizations it states: 'Links can be developed between staff and local voluntary and self-help groups. Such groups may be able to provide individual support or be invited to contribute to training in mental health awareness' (p.23). User and voluntary agencies have a range of skills and experience which can not only inform practice but also highlight needs, shape health strategy, encourage networks and highlight the significance of connections with other agencies on mental health and illness.

User involvement has implications if professional mental health staff attempt to 'do it'. It is not an easy task. Bostock (1991) examined the strengths and weaknesses of professional involvement in communities from a community psychology perspective: 'It is difficult for professionals to work without giving people in communities the impression that their suffering is not structural but individual, curable pathology'. This danger of the professionalization of human needs is one that runs through policy and the intentions of well-meaning advocates for user-friendly mental health. Systems and processes developed to engage users in consultation and modification of service provision and planning can appear manipulative, particularly to marginalized and oppressed groups. Butcher (1993) describes a shift in emphasis by the 1980s from care in the community to care by the community. This has broadened to include other population groups such as older people, people with physical disabilities and people in chronic ill-health. It is also based on assumptions that, with the appropriate resources, communities are able and willing to care for their own vulnerable members supported by a range of professional and voluntary agencies. User participation and mental health tie in with community policies that identify with the notion of the active community. They are designed to develop, maintain or draw upon the notion of the active community. All agencies and practitioners need to consider that some communities may lack an adequate infrastructure to perform such a role.

Mental health promotion

Connected to the areas of service users, discrimination, mental illness prevention and the potential for positive mental health and well-being is MHP as a force for users. The Trent Health Gain Investment Programme described above details the importance of user and consumer involvement in relation to promoting mental health, describing several goals:

1. To facilitate the empowerment of communities and individuals
2. To improve the scope for the prevention of mental ill health
3. To reduce inequalities.

A user focus is central to such an approach. Interestingly, a report by Greenoak *et al.* (1994) for the Health Education Authority that was intended to raise the debate nationally about the promotion of mental health makes no mention of the skills and experiences of mental health service users or their involvement or participation in service planning and provision. Similarly, the report by Bury *et al.* (1994) on the social perspectives of promoting mental health does not include the contribution of users' views. The often-cited work by Newton (1988) on the prevention of mental ill health also has limited content in terms of users' experiences and skills. The specialist mental health services may have moved into this territory, but it would be wrong to assume that they are always welcome. It could be argued that the cognitive, skill-focused coping and management approaches advocated by national policy, including the Health Education Authority, are failed attempts at addressing fundamental social and economic inequalities under a different label and in a different setting. Mental health promotion can simply become the new territory for health care professionals to colonize and monopolize. True empowerment requires risk taking and giving up or sharing of professional power. This is not a comfortable thing for professional mental health workers to do. Bearing this in mind, what can an MHP approach provide for past and present users of mental illness services? It can do several things. It can positively exploit state-led initiatives such as the Patients' Charter (DOH 1991) initiative to examine more than 'consumerist' approaches to services.

The Patients' Charter

Launched in 1991, the Patients' Charter was aimed at setting out a person's right to NHS care through a set of national standards. (The rights are set out in Chapter 10). In a recent review McIver and Martin (1996) highlight some of the inconsistencies within the charter and call for independent monitoring of the rights and standards set out. They also make a helpful point in terms of the soft (subjective) versus hard (objective) outcomes debate in health. At present the charter standards are measured by NHS league tables. Only some of the standards are monitored and the 'soft' standards are not monitored. However, these are ones that staff and patients' organizations and service users see as central to how a service is delivered: respect for privacy, dignity, and religious and cultural beliefs. As identified in previous chapters, such elements are the raw ingredients for our mental health to be sustained and promoted. McIver and Martin (1996) also set out guidelines in developing local patients' charters. If local charters are developed with local people they have several advantages (Box 8.4).

Box 8.4 **Advantages of local charters**

- Publicity during their development with patients and the public raises awareness of charter rights and standards and encourages local ownership
- The charter will reflect issues that concern service users and the public
- The involvement of local people in the monitoring of standards can increase public confidence in the results

(McIver and Martin 1996)

Another state-inspired initiative, Local Voices (DOH 1992b; NHSME 1992) also establishes the principle of public involvement in health purchasing and commissioning. And the recent report *Primary Care: The Future* (DOH 1996a) calls for patient and carer information and involvement. At the local authority level the Community Care Charter has become a government requirement of social services departments for implementation in 1996–1997. The charter is intended to act as a benchmark against which the quality and performance of services can be measured. Many have been developed in partnership with users and carers and place emphasis on information and consultation mechanisms. Clearly, despite their limitations, such a high-profile approach to public and user involvement allows opportunities for the practitioner to legitimate and agitate for action in this area.

Advocacy

Advocacy as both a concept and a practical tool has gained momentum within the mental health field over the last two decades (see Box 8.5). Recently an advocacy Code of Practice (Conlan *et al.* 1994) has been developed. This was informed by ten regional conferences about services held between service users and local managers under the auspices of the Mental Health Task Force. The code aims to inform and enable users and develop understanding among managers. It also attempts to clarify roles and functions and to act as a basis for training of staff and users. Linked with the advocacy movement is the concept of self-help which McCormick (1993) describes as being able to question medical definitions of health and illness and the stigma attached to illness. Such initiatives reclaim areas of normal life which have been defined as medical and reclaim decision rights for their members. In this sense the concept of power and of empowerment can be identified. It is this area of self-help which we now consider, and the role the practitioner can have in it.

Box 8.5 **Types of advocacy**

Public health advocacy: A process to overcome structural barriers to public health goals. Focus on policy at legislative, fiscal, physical and social environment level

Single-issue or crisis advocacy: Dealing with a complaint or ensuring access to a service, case conference, case review

Peer advocacy: Support for someone in a similar situation

Self-advocacy: Acting on one's own behalf or with support of a peer advocate. May involve a group (group advocacy)

Citizen advocacy: Long-term partnership between individual and advocate. Advocate usually trained. Offers practical and emotional support

Legal advocacy: Representation by an expert to help individuals or groups exercise their rights

---

Self-help groups and professionals

A comprehensive study by Wilson (1995) examined self-help groups and professionals who want to work together. As a qualitative study over two years it raises issues for a range of agencies and organizations at policy, planning and practice levels. The report uses a definition of self-help developed by the Nottingham Self-Help Team (20 Pelham Road, Sherwood Rise: registered charity no. 218776). This is significant for us given that the area of self-help in the mental illness area is well established by associations such as MIND, SANE, the National Schizophrenia Fellowship (NSF), the Manic Depression Fellowship (MDF), and sundry support groups and lobbyists.

Self help – a definition

A self-help or mutual aid group is made up of people who have personal experience of the same problem or life situation, either directly or through their family or friends. Sharing experiences enables them to give each other a unique quality of mutual support and to pool practical information and ways of coping. Groups are run by and for their members. Some self-help groups expand their activities. They may, for example, provide services for people who have the same problem or life situation; or they may campaign for change. Professionals may sometimes take part in the group in various ways, when asked to by the group.

The range of self-help initiatives is important in relation to the mental health field. Survivors Speak Out, for example, is seeking to change the mental health system at a fundamental level, whereas a local depression support group may not politicize itself in terms of the structural and economic determinants of mood but target pragmatic approaches to choices and knowledge of therapy. Wilson also differentiates between self-help groups (as in this definition) and what she terms 'professionally led support groups' (see Table 8.2).

Feature	Self-help groups	Professionally led groups	
			Table 8.2 **The features of self-help groups and professionally led support groups**
Structure	Informal	Formal	
Decision making	Participative	Hierarchical	
Main concern	Mutual support and information	Provision of services	
Source of knowledge	Through experience	Through training	
Degree of permanence	Uncertain	Long-term	
Reward for time	Better coping. Satisfaction from being helpful	Pay and status. Satisfaction from being helpful	
Resources	Volunteer help. Members' homes	Paid staff. Offices	*(continued overleaf)*

	Feature	Self-help groups	Professionally led groups
Table 8.2 **The features of self-help groups and professionally led support groups** (*continued*)	Degree of integration into structures	Low	High
	Language	Everyday	Jargon/shorthand

The advantages of being a member of a self-help group are identified as fivefold and include mutual support, information, confidence raising, an opportunity to be helpful, and influencing services. Wilson's research also identified differences in terms of how professionals assist the people they work with to get in touch with a group. Hand in hand with self-help and the 'creative tension' between acceptance and difference goes the area of effectiveness. As described in Chapter 7, policy and purchasing intentions and the 'business' and consumer orientation of care service mean that issues of evaluation for funding and credibility are more prominent. Evaluation of self-help is deemed important and a necessity. A recent study examined this issue from a mental health perspective in relation to Tranx support groups.

Evaluation and self-help

In her review of Tranx groups, Bewsher (1995) develops a practical 'toolbox' for evaluation (Box 8.6). It consists of a range of approaches for identifying group objectives through to measuring success. This method is applicable to groups initiated or supported by practitioners as well as being a useful tool for user groups.

Box 8.6 **Toolbox for self-help evaluation**

Setting and reviewing aims and objectives: What the group wants to achieve and action proposed to achieve this. It includes agreeing a philosophy and sharing this with new members and potential supporters and sponsors of the group

Making a video recording: Producing a video of a group's activities: this may include individual experiences

Health gain workshop: For people to evaluate effectiveness in terms of self-reported improvement in health and well-being

Group exercises: Holding discussion groups to review which activities of the self-help group are helpful

Group evaluation: To identify the successes and failures of the group

Group diary: To keep a record of activities such as how many people attend, issues discussed

Individual diary: To record individual experiences and feelings

Telephone contacts: Keep a written record of telephone enquiries and the progress of callers

(Bewsher 1995)

Several examples of exercises for evaluating health gains, activities and successes and failures have also been developed as part of this evaluation. It also highlights the significance of good dialogue which should be sustained between professional staff and organizations and self-help groups and their coordinators. The ability to sustain credibility without losing autonomy, and the ability to reflect critically on service provision (or lack of it) and on the appropriateness of services to care and support or to prevent mental illness and promote mental health are vital components of the self-help movement. Often their very existence demonstrates the inadequacy of a limited view of health and illness. They require champions to support and engage collaboratively with, and statutory agencies in the mental health and related fields are in a good position both to provide this and to assist with self-help-friendly methods of evaluation and audit.

The state perspective – 'Seeking Local Views'

Local authorities have a duty to consult fully with users and their carers in the drawing up and monitoring of community care plans. NHS purchasers and providers, including GPs, have a similar responsibility.

'Seeking Local Views', is a chapter in the Health of the Nation – Key Area Handbook: Mental Illness (DOH 1993a). This has user participation and involvement as its focus and echoes the sentiments of various documents such as HGIP (1994) which highlight practical steps that agencies should take in order to foster better dialogue and constructive criticism and involvement in service plans and delivery. The main aim is to encourage and facilitate better communication between service providers and people who use or have used them in order to improve service responsiveness and quality. While this is to be welcomed, it can be seen as no more than maintaining traditional service delivery. It remains important to stress that participation itself, while fulfilling normalization principles in terms of citizens' rights, should not be confused with its being a therapeutic activity. This may be an unintended outcome but should not shape the process. The Key Area also recognizes the particular needs of people with severe mental illness participating in

Do professionals want
user involvement only on
their own terms and under
their own control?

How would you support
self-help initiatives and
what support would you
require?

consultation and other user-focused processes. As with other documents generated by statutory agencies as well as mental health charities and user-focused activity, the argument for practical assistance to facilitate user involvement is highlighted. Key issues include matters such as the payment of expenses and paying them on time and discreetly, ensuring that ethnic minority communities are not doubly discriminated against, and an overall improvement in information.

We now examine examples of good practice which have mental health and users as their focus.

Good practice examples

Examples of good practice in consultation, support and training are significant and there is a wide variety of points at which practitioners can assist in their development.

Box 8.7 **Good practice example**

Building on experience: a training pack for mental health service users working as trainers, speakers and workshop facilitators (NHS Executive 1994a)

This pack was developed by the Mental Health Task Force after five training days were held across the United Kingdom and looked at themes of looking after ourselves as trainers, negotiation skills and presentation skills. The booklet is useful for establishing ground rules, planning training events, dealing with group dynamics and presenting information in a clear and practical way. It is relevant for both user and self-help groups and as a resource for anyone in the mental health field, including practitioners who require a framework to develop and deliver training. Mental health and other professionals should be making such documents available to as broad a range of user and self-help groups as possible. This also highlights the importance of developing ways and means of including users in planning training, in training itself and in ensuring that they can utilize the information and resource infrastructures that large organizations and services have at their disposal.

Practitioners should ensure that users and user groups have access to material.

Guidelines for a Local Charter for Users of Mental Health Services (NHS Executive 1994b)

These guidelines aim to use existing good practices, including developed charters, to produce a document relevant to a user perspective and adaptable to local needs. It is useful to examine how the framework can be used as it exemplifies the possibility of such an approach having relevance to purchasers, providers and users. It highlights how strategy, training and other initiatives can be taken on board by the respective agencies and groups. In this way MHP can also be deemed relevant to these three:

- **Purchasers** set standards for all service contracts
- **Providers** improve the quality of the service
- **Service user groups** negotiate with purchasers and providers

Key themes that make up the framework include:

- Personal dignity and respect
- Information
- Accessibility
- Participation and involvement
- Choice
- Advocacy
- Confidentiality and records
- Complaints
- Treatment
- The Mental Health Act 1993

A summary of rights is included in Chapter 10. Elements of these are also reflected in the Butterworth review as examined in Chapter 2 and by Boxer and McCulloch (1996). As discussed in Chapter 2 on the role of policy and its implications for MHP, the recent review of mental health nursing also stresses the importance of a user focus beyond the professional carer intervention. Two recommendations are most significant in terms of the user movement. Recommendation 1 explores the whole area of culturally appropriate services. The second recommendation is key in that it sees the nurse as having a central role in ensuring that people in their care have access to appropriate (although this is never defined) information, including treatment options and rights.

The Butterworth Report (Butterworth 1994) recommends that people who use mental health services and their carers should participate in teaching and curriculum development. What evidence do you have for such involvement in your training experience? How might you encourage such an approach?

It is essential that practitioners utilize the documents and guidelines described. However, the process should be more than a tick-box for the convenience of mental health and related services. If it is to work it requires shifts in both thinking and practices to more user- and consumer-orientated ones. Another document, by Anglia and Oxford Regional Health Authority (1994), places users and carers as the final chapter in the review and suggests three levels of involvement: the individual, project and district levels. They also provide examples of initiatives aimed at involving users and carers, including employing a worker to assist in the transition from hospital to community-based services and use of formal surveys of current and past users.

Box 8.8 Good practice example: *Direct Power*

Leader (1995) has developed a Direct Power pack for people who want to develop their support networks and a personalized plan of care. This refutes the professional notion of 'management' of care and the view that people reject or refuse services as a result of their mental distress. Instead such refusal of service is seen as having more to do with services which are oppressive, are not individual, and sustain dependency. The pack provides information about community care and enables the individual to work through an assessment of their needs in order to build up a care plan. The pack contains guidelines for building a personal profile and a current circumstances checklist, and covers experiences of services used or being used, a self-assessment of needs, help and support contacts, partnership agreements and hospital and discharge arrangements. Even more relevant for this chapter is the inclusion of notes for mental health workers to encourage empowerment of clients they are in contact with.

Practitioners should examine this and similar material and familiarize themselves with a philosophy and practice which has the user – and the potential user – at the forefront

---

Conclusion

We have a progression in relation to the involvement of users of mental illness and mental health services having a say in how they are treated (in the broadest sense as well as the clinical) from the statements of the World Health Organization, to statutory service purchasers and providers, to the user movement and its allies. The emphasis on a market economy approach to health and social care determining a range of other possibilities may quicken the pledging and giving of resources in order to make true user participation a reality. One key point to emerge in much of the literature is that the efforts of users and advocates to 'tackle' the system have been made more difficult by the NHS reforms that were intended in part to improve user involvement. Structures, systems, language and personalities have all been replaced. Ironically, what is often on offer is a willingness for dialogue between the new world order and the old battle-scarred survivors. It is little wonder that they find it tough. This is made more difficult when there is a professional assumption that the user movement will drop everything else it is trying to do (with little help or resources) and head for the tables of health care providers and purchasers of mental health provision. The failure by District Health Authorities and Mental Health Service managers and their staff to extend their consultation systems into the worlds of mental health service users may result in another form of exclusion and fulfil negative prophecies of user reluctance, stubbornness or inability. All is not lost. The needs of the bureaucracy itself in terms of pledges and policies in a whole series of governmental documents mean that the user's voice is here to stay. Ostensibly, user participation, collaboration or involvement is power sharing, or power education by the systems and structures of mental health purchasers and providers. As such, there is a learning journey that needs to take place and which we all need to be on.

Practice checklist

- Become familiar with the literature and material relating to the user movement.

- Acknowledge and appreciate the tension between your role as a practitioner and supporter/enabler of user initiatives.

- Support can consist of taking user participation seriously, offering a venue, administrative support, information on other services and agencies.

- As a practitioner you are unlikely to be a user yourself: respect the wishes for users doing it their way.

- Champion the cause. Disseminate user-led practice, projects and ideas.

- Offer your skills and experience – do not impose them upon a group or an individual.

- Exploit existing mechanisms such as charters, participation strategies and stakeholder approaches to take forward a user perspective.

- Encourage user involvement in training initiatives.

9

Conclusions and recommendations

Promotion of mental health is a worthy cause. It is a doable task, a necessary ingredient of action that may be undertaken to make our world progress, to help humanity survive as a society of humans rather than as an assembly of creatures striving to live unaware of themselves and of the links which tie them to their past, their futures and those around them. (Sartorious 1996)

Key themes:

- Areas of debate
- Public, professionals and the state
- Informing ourselves

Overview

In this chapter we draw together key elements of MHP from other chapters and further identify why we think a framework for practice is so important in this field. We recognize that there are no tablets of stone; each individual or group of people within a specific locality will be as much governed by personal and economic motivation and constraints, as we are in attempting to move mental health practice into the twenty-first century, by addressing mental health promotion as more than rhetoric. Our mental health is also a private matter in the order of things and at no time have we, in personal, academic and practice terms, lost sight of the fact that however much health might be at the top of a lot of people's most-wanted list, for others it might not. As health becomes more and more of a commodity for some and an unattainable necessity for others, for example the massive growth in cosmetic surgery and the difficulty in obtaining organs for donation, representation of health in its widest context has been considered throughout our account.

In our introduction we identified the elements of the public, health and social care professionals, and the state as the foundation for developing practice for MHP. We have addressed these broad themes throughout the book as well as more specific evaluation and examples of practice in areas ranging from hospital to community-focused care, user involvement and education. We have clearly identified the problems with any over-determined definitions of mental health and illness and have provided further reading and critique of this highly important but complex area of understanding. We have clarified that from our perspective MHP is the action element missing in much of current mainstream mental health practice and we hope that among students and fellow colleagues there is at least a commitment to explore this further.

At a statutory level, in our analysis, we have identified that certain government policies, especially in the form of the National Health Strategy: Health of the Nation, have inspired a degree of legitimacy in the area of MHP. Despite its limitations, it has allowed a range of stakeholders in purchasing and service provision for mental illness services to construct viable responses to a host of actions which have explicitly included MHP. As can be shown in Table 9.1, the influences cover the span of specialist and noninstitutional responses to mental health as much as to mental illness. While we would welcome broader inclusion of MHP, rather than a limited preventive and educational focus on 'educating the public' to understand mental illness, its interpretation in state policy remains incomplete. For example, the workplace as a MHP setting is a convenient 'laboratory' in which to exercise stress management approaches to structural inadequacy. We would argue this has to be more comprehensive and that there is room for innovation and agenda setting for the MHP practitioner. It is this aspect of the role of the MHP practitioner that we will go on to discuss in more detail. It is, after all, a role that many statutory and informal agencies can and do work to.

Aims	Actions	
		Table 9.1 **Responses to mental health/illness**
Mental health promotion	NHS and local authority workplace Prevention strategies in workplace Health promotion in schools, housing, media, etc.	
Caring for mentally ill offenders	Diversion from the criminal justice system	
Developing comprehensive services	Providing care in the community Replacing old institutions Care programmes	
Improving information	Outcomes: standardized assessments Auditing suicide Supervision registers	
Alliances and joint purchasing	Joint purchasing of mental health services	*(continued overleaf)*

Table 9.1 **Responses to mental health/illness** (*continued*)	**Aims**	**Actions**
		Coordination between primary and secondary care Involving users and carers
	Improving training, education and good practice	Improving the recognition of depression, anxiety and suicide Reducing use of benzodiazepines Development of good practice guidelines

Areas of debate 1

A 'menu' approach

As with the example given in Table 9.1, we acknowledge that a 'menu' approach to the issues of mental illness care, treatment, education and prevention and the promotion of mental health could be viewed as too simplistic. In exploring these elements we have tried to define and identify boundaries and highlight where successes and failures, at the level of professional and ideological understanding and involvement, meet with reality, and to show how these approaches arise. It would appear from undertaking literature reviews related to each of the chapters in the book, that they could be the subject matter of a book in their own right.

Despite obvious limitations, a menu approach does provide us with a range of choices in terms of interventions, models and viewpoints. This can enable a more critical decision-making process and highlight areas in which further choice should be made, or clarify why a choice is made. This in itself is as enlightening, empowering and ultimately mental health-promoting as more traditional approaches to the subject.

Individuality

Why is there so much emphasis on individualized focused approaches, with their basis in preventive education or a very limited notion of healing? Tudor (1996) provides a useful synopsis of the work of Jennifer Newton in highlighting the problems of this approach, as we have done in Chapter 6, and this is an important area of debate. Obviously, the problems of this approach may be the ones that sit more comfortably with a particular professional intervention in health and social care provision, but they reside within culture and practice and have a powerful function in maintaining the status quo of 'us' and 'them', especially through the creation of elitist language and misplaced ideological vision. Choice may be limited, and dependent on many complex variables, but creative as well as reflective practice has to be considered. We have explored ways in which this is being and could be achieved throughout this book.

Representation

The media are perhaps the main vehicle with which to identify and analyse whether people do understand that they can effect change, often at a relatively minor level, which can constantly impact on both individual and collective mental health. There is very little current research available with which to disseminate mental health promotion strategies, and only one example of intervention at international level from current CD-Rom searches. MIND, in respect of its policy statements and in *OpenMind*, continually tries to raise and maintain the profile of mental health issues and MHP, but it is a shame that the general public do not see this as a mainstream journal. The emerging psychotherapy/counselling approaches and alternative/complementary therapies are perhaps two areas in which our ideas about health do not carry the same correlation between physical and mental illness, and they have gone a long way in changing attitudes about health and the precursors of major mental illnesses, from sexual abuse to food allergies.

Media portrayal of mental health and illness in this country usually concentrates on negative reinforcement of the latter. Very little public involvement in this subject takes place, apart from soul-searching chat shows and the occasional documentary or realistic drama. News coverage of recent tragedies concerning the mentally ill do nothing to illuminate a public already anxious about the mental health state of their neighbours and whose recourse is to want conformation of diagnosis and exclusion from social life (Barham and Hayward 1995). The mentally ill have always been a useful scapegoat for the ills of this society, when, in statistical terms, we know that it is our family and friends who do us the most harm. This is further highlighted in a study undertaken in Scotland which examined various media representations of the mentally ill (Philo *et al.* 1992).

Negation

However much we have stressed the importance of user involvement, or identified how this is at the core of our realization of mental health promotion, it would be naive to presume that this is anything more than touching the proverbial tip of the iceberg. Inequality in mental health services is not diminishing, and at the time of writing this book the continued campaign against racism and sexism is still nowhere near being resolved. The overuse of medication as front-line treatment for all manner of problems still gives cause for alarm. The recent changes to the Mental Health Act 1985, such as the delicately rephrased 'aftercare with supervision' amendment (1996), do nothing to allay public concern about the mentally ill and the need for containment, rather than appropriate services being developed to cover a wide spectrum of problems. The persistent call for more hospital beds goes against any research findings that, whatever the problems with community care, those leaving more formal statutory institutions do not want to return to them or to be treated as they have been in them. Since September 1996 care in the community has been renamed 'comprehensive mental health services', presumably to obviate the problem by changing language rather than attitude or economic investment, and therefore to vitiate the impact it has had both negatively and positively. This would seem to be a similar ploy to that used by politicians in other key aspects of our lives, and as realized in current debates around political correctness. If something has become too sensitive, alter a word or phrase: henceforth there are no fundamental problems with care in the community; nor do black people have any problem with racism, or racist language, they are just perpetrating an ideological myth with no foundation whatsoever in language. In this way we never escape the past or arrive at a more comprehensive and equitable future, and the onus on individual accountability and responsibility remains confused, if not corrupt.

Exclusion

In further identifying how language is so important, we can highlight the term 'vulnerable' with its various negative connotations and its links to a traditional programme development for the most 'deserving'. With the continual erosion of welfare provision, and yet another alarming financial crisis in the health service at the time of writing this book, the services for those already labelled as having a serious or enduring mental illness become more tenuous. The use of the term 'worried well' has not been mentioned so far but, as with political correctness, by its use the underlying problem is masked by whoever has a vested interest in doing so – and for the mentally ill there are many key players. The decision to extend the tentacles of the Mental Health Act, for example the discussion document 'Mentally Disordered Offenders: Sentencing and Discharge Arrangements', can only further detract from any real emphasis given to positive mental health.

In an article in *OpenMind* entitled 'Horrible Hybrids', Harrison (1996) makes two very important points related to the proposed change to make a hospital order run concurrently with a prison sentence. If hospital treatment ends before the fixed sentence, transfer would be to continue the remainder of it in prison, in line with the need to protect the public and to punish offenders, whether they have a mental illness or not. This is a punitive element to care of the mentally ill as it brings in the notion of responsibility and retribution, and has little to do with the primary focus of causation and treatment of mental illness, let alone allowing for someone to have their mental health needs acknowledged.

MIND has published written accounts from people who say they would rather be in prison than in hospital as the latter often represents a much more covert way of removing people from society permanently:

> . . . they are not as closely watched, they cannot be treated against their will, and they are more likely to know when they will be released. When our prisons can be such terrible places, what does that say about our hospitals? People sent to hospital by the courts usually spend longer there than they would in prison. The hospital order is indeterminate . . . and most restriction orders are made without limit of time . . . So, the power to detain indefinitely to protect the public from a 'mentally disordered offender' already exists.' (Harrison 1996, p.13)

Investment

The rapid growth in the private sector of mental illness provision as well as the prison service means that those without any economic power have no say in where, how, and for how long they are 'treated' in this domain if the cost represents lower or higher profits for private employers. There is a time-bomb ticking away, not only in private provision but in underfunded local authority dwellings where large numbers of care assistants and unqualified staff are expected to perform miracles, often for less than £3 per hour and with very little available support from the few qualified staff accountable for them. What does this say about the priority given to mental health issues, especially in terms of long-term care for the seriously or chronically disabled and particularly older adults? Unless we see this as everybody's business, and consider that it involves something more than short-term gain, we could all find ourselves at some time in our life seeking mental health care and realizing its deficiencies too late. MIND's latest figures show a massive increase, not a decline, in those seeking psychiatric assessment and treatment. Overburdened communities and community mental health teams cannot or should not undertake to put right the damage done by punitive legislation, instant gratification and neglect. If change cannot be effected by strategic policies because economic investment is misplaced or lacking, then no matter how strong people are in coping with the obstacles, or being imaginative in how care programmes are implemented, stress and burnout become major factors for all parties involved. If this is the defining element of empathic and collaborative practice between users of services and those who work for them, perhaps it has to get to crisis point to effect change at the level necessary. There is a real shortage of mental health nurses at present and no shortage of jobs. The enormity of the task can very quickly turn around the best intentions of anyone working in this field, and it is not surprising that misplaced investment, entrenched attitudes and bad practice cannot be altered as quickly as many people would hope.

Collaboration

We also need to consider the extent to which we can construct a framework that is applicable. After all, there is inherent conflict between the needs of purchasers and policy makers, service providers and users. This tension is important – it is what moves things on as well as holds us back. Such a framework can only highlight opportunities and look forward. As ever, there are no easy answers and few simple solutions, but there are ways of doing things and doing them better. Hornby (1993), in her book about collaborative practice, identifies what skills are required, and how they could be put to best effect (p.161). Most importantly of all, especially in the role of public service, there is considerable scope to improve our understanding of mental health at little extra cost, and motivational factors cannot be ignored. For the first time the public as well as 'professionals' have the chance to enrol on courses which address mental health from the perspective we would consider most important. The Open University now has one course beginning in 1997 which would seem to underpin the points we raise, in a truly collaborative sense, with people experiencing problems. The course is entitled 'Mental Health and Distress: Perspectives and Practice; and supported by a text from service users' viewpoints (Read and Reynolds 1996).

A recent initiative from Northern Ireland 'Working Together: A Focus on Health and Social Well-being' (1996) concerning all community nurses has been to put into action a vision of working together which goes way beyond the boundaries of how care is being undertaken in Britain. The emphasis is on user involvement at all levels, but most importantly nurses will have to provide evidence of this collaboration in fourteen identified target areas, and the commitment given primarily to seeing health in its political and social context must be accepted by all involved, including managers. In this respect the broadening out of what constitutes mental health promotion should not dilute its impact, and this highlights a crucial role for mental health nursing within the social domain not adequately recognized in traditional nursing education to date (Working Together: A Focus on Health and Social Well-Being; NIDHSSS 1996).

The findings of the Butterworth Report (1994), with its emphasis on 'working in partnership' had already identified some of the main problems and solutions to effective mental health practice. It would seem Project 2000 is not able to meet the needs of mental health nurse education and practice; and the needs of working within the domain of mental health and illness in complex social and cultural settings. This is also problematic in terms of the expectations of being able to treat the mentally ill in the community without changing attitudes and values about people in the broadest sense of life experience (Barker *et al.* 1997).

Working with, not for others

At the level of practice involvement, we hope that this book can be of value as much to 'nonprofessionals' as it is to those who feel they have a strategic professional role. Examples of 'good practice' have been identified wherever possible, but we realize that at the time of writing this is still an emerging perspective and we apologize for any omissions in highlighting work being undertaken in this country and farther afield. The development of mental health and social care provision in Canada is a good example of how parallel activities are taking place within this discipline (Austin *et al.* 1996). There will be those who might question how, conceptually, notions of mental health and anti-oppressive practice can be integrated, as exemplified in the arguments surrounding the 'correct' theoretical basis of mental health nursing and social work. Is it primarily psychology, or sociology, or both, or do we consider more closely the physical, psychological and social domains and see theory development as a gradual process, dependent on many factors?

We have also discussed the emergence of anti-oppressive practice as the core element on which the rest of our competence and scope for practice and action develop. This is vital before one thinks of oneself as an expert in psychological and social dynamics. We would hope that whatever perceptions there are of concepts such as oppression and empowerment, they only enrich understanding and do not negate it (Humphries 1996). Further reading in this area has been indicated where appropriate and underpins many of the issues we have raised. Other sources of insight exist in many forms: media, literature, music, art, poetry, oral history, dialogue, and personal acknowledgement of our own mental health needs and problems.

Action

For students and 'survivors' of the psychiatric system, we hope that this book will encourage you to take more of an active part in this aspect of mental health practice. Incorporating mental health promotion as another core element of health and social care education is not easy, for the reasons we have discussed. A framework for mental health promotion has also to address the needs of learners and practitioners at all levels, but we are acutely aware that major change in education and training within the context of mental health practice is still undetermined and paradoxical in its approach and parameters. We have taken a different approach from Tudor's recent book, as the only other benchmark in this field, and in key chapters have tried to show more explicitly the practical necessity of mental health promotion in the intertwining of people, professionals and the state. At the same time we acknowledge the philosophical reflection inherent in this subject and end this section with what can only be a partial account to date. Much more thought, dialogue and action is needed and, in the words of Paulo Friere, we know it will come, since any society or 'community' changes, adapts, integrates, fragments. That is the nature of the dialectic of experience and learning:

> We have to recognize, in a first approach to the subject, how difficult it is for us to 'walk the streets of history' – regardless of whether we 'step back' from practice in order to theorize it, or are engaged in it – succumbing to the temptation either to over-estimate our objectivity and reduce consciousness to it, or to discern or understand consciousness as the almighty maker and arbitrary re-maker of the world . . . . Subjectivism or mechanistic objectivism are both antidialectical, and thereby incapable of apprehending the permanent tension between consciousness and the world . . . . It is only in a dialectical perspective that we grasp the role of consciousness in history, disentangled from any distortion that either exaggerates its importance or cancels, rejects it. (Friere 1996, p.100)

Areas of debate 2

In this section we address more specifically the role of the public, professionals and the state in bringing together the key elements of our framework for MHP. We considered an approach in Chapter 5 which would require that the identification of comprehensive practice resides in being more forward thinking in the social domain than has been the case so far, especially in mental health nursing.

The public

> In both lay and professional thinking, mental illness has usually been viewed as the property of isolated individuals – it is people who are 'mad', not families or community groupings, still less whole societies. The origin of such illness, however, is not necessarily to be located in such individuals – though that is by far and away the most popular assumption. In fact the

supposition that psychiatric disorder might have an extra-personal as well as personal psychological dimension emerged in twentieth century psychiatry through a slow and piecemeal process. (Prior 1993, p.111)

Within the public domain, government and 'professional' rhetoric only serves to confuse a very mixed population of people bombarded on all sides by the necessity of life in the late twentieth century. Exposures of our most basic instincts have become so commonplace that there is ever more blurring between fantasy and reality. The link is especially tenuous within the confines of deprivation, abuse and violence in familial relationships. This is our basic start in life, living in a family or with carers who are supposed to nurture our physical, emotional, spiritual and cultural needs. There are so many testaments to how this goes or has gone wrong that this subject alone could engage us in study for the rest of our lives, as it has so many eminent theorists. The need for sustained loving relationships is paramount in our society. Marriage is still the symbolic union to counter isolation and to secure needs and wants at all levels. Considering that this country has the highest divorce rate in Western Europe, the pressure on people to conform to public expectations somehow does not measure up with the reality of experience. Isolation and loneliness foster so many problems that many of the patients using psychiatric services are being forced to say that they are ill to gain some appropriate human contact, and to get away from abusive, violent and neglectful situations. Sadly, these experiences often continue within the psychiatric system. If we are to change our attitudes and investment in health and emotional well-being, it has been obvious for a long time, and from many different theoretical accounts which agree at this point, that this needs to start at a very early age. There are very few areas in the country committed to tackling mental health issues in this way. Hackney is one of the only boroughs to have a mental health promotion worker funded by the health authority and working in schools not only to develop antibullying approaches but to consider the enormous strain and uncertainty placed on younger people in all aspects of social integration and multifaceted cultural and religious existence. The call by the widow of Stephen Lawrence for a 'moral referendum' to stem the tide of violence and 'bad behaviour', by introducing something akin to a public 'code of conduct', has captured the imagination of many people. Unless the priority given to both individual and community mental health is increased, expecting the public to solve the problems with which 'experts' have seemingly had little success might end up as more hollow words.

Public involvement

. . . If we are able to acknowledge our isolated situations in existence and to confront them with resoluteness, we will be able to turn lovingly toward others. If on the other hand, we are overcome with dread before the abyss of loneliness, we will not reach out toward others but instead will flail at them in order not to drown in the sea of existence. In this instance our relationships will not be true relationships at all, but out of joint miscarriages, distortions of what might have been. (Yalom 1980, p.363)

How can people become involved in and be able to understand the importance of mental health promotion in countering all the obstacles put in the way by ourselves as individuals, who make up this public, and the professionals and politicians we become, or who think they know better, and in whom we then invest power and trust? Community development and participation are considered to be the bridges linking professional awareness and involvement with locally identified needs. Unfortunately, this has to be underpinned by government strategies at national level in terms of funding and sets precedents about what kinds of interventions have value. Equally complex is the moral issue of earning money from human distress without considering that some kind of reparation might be necessary. Some active role is necessary, and at the level of community participation can bring a sense of realism to the very 'unreal' world of the mental institution.

The key players in the voluntary sector currently have an especially difficult role to fulfil, and lack of funding in this sector can often bring to the fore crucial concerns. Public investment in charities and voluntary organizations has suffered from the introduction of the national lottery, and by the increased need to justify the 'cause'. If a charitable organization like the National Lifeboat Institute can have over £200 million sitting in the bank, while other organizations will not get any mainstream funding or public support because they are not 'neutral' or do not play at the heart strings of the moral majority, as people with mental health problems do not, what hope is there in resolving the acute contradictions which exist in terms of the role the public plays in this? This is without going back over the notion of charitable contribution and the role it plays in maintaining economic and class-based inequalities.

The main problem might be that the more 'professional' people become, the less they have in common with the needs and wants of those in their care, or their neighbours and local community. To become bound to the language systems which operate in health and social care, only to read the 'right' books, journals and newspapers, and to lose sight of the painful reality of 'lived' experience through the major psychological defence of intellectualization can isolate and obscure very 'real' issues. Working with people who have mental health problems is probably one of the most difficult and taxing of jobs, as the statistics for suicide and mental health problems among psychiatrists, nurses, social workers and other therapists confirm. Involvement with people outside of work, either in one's family, socially or in terms of community involvement, can bring about many pressures on individuals to be all things to all people. Public perceptions of mental health and illness are slow to change and as we become more burdened by economic necessity there is not the time, inclination or patience to alter misconceived notions of madness or to really have the skills and ability to confront the trauma of bereavement, abuse, violence, and oppression, unless personal experience necessitates this. The paradox that we live with as social beings can only be ignored for so long, and the more people admit to not being able to cope the more open the discussions can be about what it is that afflicts us all, both physically and mentally. It might then be possible to find more collaborative ways to work with people and to remove artificial boundaries in terms of needs and wants and assessment of these (Leader 1995).

The development of self-help/community groups has been mentioned as a very obvious way that mental health promotion functions, and it would be useful if there were more material available to show how people support each other more informally. Consideration of the diversity within our cultural life has focused where possible on highlighting the provision, or lack of it, for those from different ethnic backgrounds and also the impact of a more mixed cultural existence which has developed in different parts of the country. The more people can find common bonds within their cultural beliefs and apply them to living where they do, the more can be achieved in the quest for equitable social participation; partly because people's own needs and wants are then being addressed, but fundamentally because they are free of the shackles of racism, prejudice, and bigotry so detrimental to one's mental health state. Issues of race are also intertwined, for example, with gender identity, age, disability; and the scope for developing services for 'minority' experience, whether as a white person or black person, is still steeped in notions of the 'other' and confusion of our needs as a 'whole' person.

This would be the starting point for mental health promotion – to address the mental health needs of a given population in terms of primarily public experience and debate, rather than to preach the message of some of the more unattainable targets of Health for All. The levels of deprivation and the inequality that pervades life in Britain make this a very difficult task. However little has been stressed about the moral or ethical dimension of mental health promotion, the same principles and dilemmas apply as in relation to all aspects of mental health practice from the perspective of the past, present and future. It is important to consider this at many levels of analysis and debate, especially in terms of our being able to balance the need for rationality with emotive response in the public as well as the private arena.

Professionals

> Psychiatry is not an unambiguous instrument of good-will from all standpoints . . . changes and liberalizations of psychiatric thought have not influenced public conceptions of what psychiatry is about; only mental health professionals have seen these changes. The trick, as in the story of the Emperor's new suit of clothes, is to know what you are going to see and only then will you 'see it'. Insiders to professional codes and practices see revolutions in thought and humanization in practice where every person sees problems of morality, propriety, offensive conduct, bunches of keys, asylum walls, and danger. (Pearson 1975, p.16)

Current thinking within the domain of mental health practice is very difficult to conceptualize as a whole. Increasingly, professionals are caught up in a process of containment. This is based on clinical and financial decisions, in terms of predominantly health needs, and now a necessity to enlist any support for those experiencing psychological and social problems. Is it better to live with the stigma of being labelled mentally ill, and categorized at the highest level of the care programme approach, or to have one's needs continually ignored or deprioritized? The emphasis of this book has been at no time to couch reality in 'ethereal' terms, but to consider a variety of ways that professionals can take the lead in being able to promote mental health. There is still not enough evidence that the major mental illnesses can be cured, and that still leaves an individual with their unique set of problems and experiences. Who will, no matter what the label, require understanding and some positive action from professionals to assist them to cope with this, however it is labelled or defined.

Diverse opinions are very apparent, not only between the positions adopted by key players at the level of education and training in psychiatry, mental health nursing and social work, but also in terms of standards for provision and practice within the diversity of care facilities available. At the time of writing this book, current nursing journals provide evidence of great polarization in our understanding of the nature and treatment of 'madness'. Is it possible to accept the importance of diagnosis, or even dual-diagnosis, if that then places human response in such limited and categorical terms, to be treated primarily by a pill? Or is it just too difficult and tempting of psychological damage to journey through the philosophical and critical social theory debates to arrive at the only possible answer – that there isn't one, just a lot of very seductive ideas and theories which might not be of much use in the rehabilitation ward for sex offenders in a special hospital?

Fundamentally there has to be a basis for action which accepts, as we have highlighted, the need for consensus about what constitutes positive mental health and an attempt to encourage strategies to enable this. If this means that there has to be much closer examination of personal dynamics or the development of self-awareness, then ways should be found to support this. As many nurses and social workers are now training as counsellors, it might seem timely not to have to wait until the end of a three-year intensive course to attain much of what counselling training offers as a framework and a way of practice (Lago and Thompson 1996). We write this at a time when counselling services are being contracted because cash-starved health and local authorities cannot meet the basic requirements of the care programme approach. Therapeutic intervention by professionals is increasingly seen as a luxury, and our work in the field would confirm that it is the voluntary sector which ends up with unreasonable demands placed on it by being caught up in an artificial purchaser and providers split in welfare provision. The statutory services that offer psychotherapy and counselling are inundated with referrals and have long waiting lists. There is also a hardening of attitude by local authority managers, and it is becoming clear that the main function of mental health social workers is to carry out basic social care needs assessment. The opportunity for everyone in community mental health teams to identify therapeutic practice, and to co-ordinate care plans cannot be realized because of the acute crisis in in-patient services and the increasing number of statutory duties that have to be met.

The necessity of understanding the mechanisms which support legislation and the development of political relationships as well as therapeutic ones has to be considered an equally important, but to date essentially a neglected, part of nurse training. Knowledge and understanding within the domain of community practice would seem to be the most positive professional link to health and social care provision. Obviously, this has to be seen as part of a broader educational canvas that has to range from strategies in infant schools to the development of life-long learning, as with the University of the Third Age, and this again highlights the interdependence of health and education. If people were encouraged to develop their interpersonal skills from the earliest age, it might encourage more openness and dialogue which could take place in a variety of settings, and not just for 50 minutes as part of an artificial psychodynamic process. The elitism that is fostered because of the barrier that professional language puts up, belies the pragmatic realization that what is needed is usually very practical and based in common sense, not highly elaborate interpretation. Housing services have always played a major role in determining how a lot of people live together; increasingly they are responsible for the care of the mentally ill in the community. The boundaries that define professional status are becoming blurred, at the same time as the monolithic structure of the health service further fragments, and care is further diversified and costed.

Points to consider

The teaching of mental health promotion, if linked to therapeutic endeavour, would seem to be subsumed by the creation of individual 'experts' vying for territory.

If linked to the vast field of health promotion and education as a whole, it becomes easily diluted in its impact on people's lives.

If it exists in a political arena, whether internationally, nationally and locally, it becomes a threat to different power bases and consequentially, elitist or traditionalist approaches.

Perhaps the hardest lesson to learn, if professional status has to be the desired goal, is how to acquire more understanding and involvement in what is meant by being 'professional' and how we become or remain 'authentic' in this domain, no better or no worse than others.

The state

> 'The state is not . . . separate from us, a 'thing' remote and monolithic, devoid of contradictions. Rather in its 'extended form' it penetrates into every possible sphere of social relations, attempting to establish them as fields of its power. The contemporary crisis of the city, the socio-political disaffiliation of so many of its inhabitants, and the absence of hegemonic apparatus for their incorporation, make it obligatory for the state to establish authority – beyond purely repressive forms. (Craig *et al.* 1982)

Recent policy statements and approaches taken by the main political parties indicate the need for consideration at the level of ideology to be more acute than ever. Any shift to the 'right' or the 'left' for the purposes of securing research funding or academic glory, or winning a general election, detracts from the expressed need for collaboration, partnership and participation that we have stressed as necessary for effective mental health promotion. The portrayal of 'New Labour', in 1996 is of a party having to distance itself from the core values of socialism and further dilute the notion of 'working with people in care' (Barker *et al.* 1996). In terms of our understanding of the part that social justice plays in supporting the very fabric of democratic existence, it is questionable whether the welfare of all but the most disadvantaged will be realistically encouraged and supported whichever political party is in power (Dominelli 1997a).

Economically, the bottomless pits of health and education, by their very nature, undermine much of what mental health promotion tries to address. The rhetoric of a long line of Conservative health ministers has been to justify the closure of hospitals and reduction in hospital bed numbers while at the same time stating, at an ideological level, that it is the best course of action to intern people who can fit more and more easily into numerous categories of 'mad' or 'bad'. The rise in the numbers of secure units and the higher profile given to forensic psychiatry has meant that the investment of money in primary intervention has been diverted, and it is at local level where information can be gained as to what mental health-promoting strategies are being developed in this complex field. The massive growth in the private sector of mental health care has in most cases also been a testament to the power of monetarism, rather than any therapeutic process. Research and monitoring of this aspect of mental health care is tenuous and uncoordinated. Government charters that have raised the profile of rights and responsibilities have given false hope to thousands of people caught up in an artificial divide between health and social care needs assessment. The crux for any of the main political parties would seem to be an overdue re-examination of political values, and students might consider this an important starting point in exploring a theoretical framework to practice in health and social care.

The need to consider mental health promotion within the sphere of political activity is undeniable, and an informed understanding of the impact of social policy and state intervention, especially from the perspective of social history and social policy, is a necessary but overlooked aspect of nursing education. Evaluation and research are also overdue, in raising the profile of mental health promotion and in deciding how it might be incorporated into mainstream practice rather than being seen as the icing on the cake or part of some covert measure stemming from the Health of the Nation initiative in its support for self-individuation.

There is no one approach taken by the main political parties which goes anywhere near establishing whether the National Health Service will survive as a public institution, and we write this account with the understanding that the welfare state is up for grabs. Such basic issues as deprivation and poverty overarch any specific identification of mental health or illness that we have covered or that has been addressed elsewhere. The main concern, in terms of quelling public unease about the numbers of homicides and suicides, concentrates political rhetoric on ridding ourselves of this problem, with no real commitment by anyone to examining our mental health needs.

Whichever political party governs this country as we move towards the year 2000, the stark choices that have to be faced about cost and rationing of resources are not going to go away. If the NHS becomes a two-tier service, it is apparent that the majority of people we have considered in our account might not even be affected by this. Their needs are predominantly in the social domain, which really does challenge society's, politicians' and 'professional's' belief systems and values about 'caring' for people rather than treating illness.

Some final thoughts

> Perhaps it requires such depths of oppression to create heights of character
> . . . . I always knew that deep down in the human heart, there was mercy
> and generosity. No one is born hating another person because of the colour
> of his skin, or his background, or his religion. People must learn to hate,
> and if they can learn to hate, they can be taught to love, for love comes
> more naturally to the human heart than its opposite. (Nelson Mandela
> 1994, p.615)

Finally, we need to reiterate how important it is to be clear about the
foundation of mental health promotion. We have considered the
dichotomies inherent within current approaches to mainstream practice and identified our rationale for at least considering an approach to
our mental health needs and wants that is primarily about socioeconomic 'lived' experience. This experience is so vast, so personal, that to
presume a major change at this level or in any theoretical paradigm
shift is idealistic if we consider the experience of billions of people
from a global perspective. In other chapters in this book we have tried
to identify different projects, resources and examples of good practice.
This has been difficult to achieve from an international perspective. We
are aware of initiatives in Canada and Europe but, because of differences in identified roles and structure, this is another main area for
further research and development (Austin *et al.* 1996). Other perspectives are also realized from considering health education and promotion
more generally; this is a valid approach, but it can mean that all too
easily our mental health needs become subsumed by other agendas,
whereas we consider they are paramount. There is an enormous range
of perspectives which determine professional involvement in mental
health promotion. In the late 1990s we are seeing such developments
as the rise of the 'housing association' and the private sector as two of
the key players in people's welfare needs. The indications are that
profit, not the physical, psychological and social-environmental needs
and wants of any given neighbourhood or community, is the main
concern; and that training opportunities will be piecemeal and inadequate in terms of the spectrum that education and training now encom-
passes (MIND 1995). At the same time we are seeing more public and
interagency involvement. In early 1996 the Anglican Church held its
first open referendum on poverty, including those people who are
experiencing a level of poverty and deprivation not seen for a long time,
in the hope that a more collaborative way could be found to address
the negative social and individual life experience in 'modern' Britain.
Very often it is individual people, forced into the limelight because of
personal tragedy which mirrors the worst nightmare scenarios of us all,

who can change public, professionals' and the state's involvement. Mental health promotion spans the need for rational thinking and planning, but hopefully identifies the emotional or intuitive aspects of human relationships.

From our understanding, both professionally and personally, there will always be the paradox of numerous people who are mentally healthy and playing an active role in promoting their lives and the lives of those around them but who have survived the worst experiences anyone could imagine having to face. This book should be dedicated to them. In the introductory chapter we identified some of the factors which underpin positive mental health, and in Chapter 5 we considered this in terms of user-led approaches or involvement in the education and training agenda. We would ask you to reconsider this in the light of what you have read. The impetus to consider MHP as something intrinsic to the way we behave towards and interact with others is vital and still probably the most neglected aspect. We have stressed that the link between MHP and anti-oppressive practice, feminist practice and humanistic/holistic approaches to health, rather than traditional and mainstream ones, can better inform who we are as human beings and the 'professionals' we might wish to become. We have tried to show our willingness to engage with others about this subject. As white 'professionals' we have, we hope, not presumed to talk for our black colleagues and users of services in this field, and not negated either individual or collective experience of living in a racist and oppressive society. Neither are we carrying around half-baked notions of madness and how to 'treat' it; our aim in writing this book is not to support those looking for scientific 'proof' or professional status before they will do something about the obvious. By concentrating on the 'madness' of others, students, practitioners, policy makers and the public find themselves entrenched in 'them and us' scenarios. In researching for this book we have, at times, been dismayed at the level of ignorance and inept communication which pervades the world of mental health and illness. Failings at an individual level cannot all be blamed on the 'system'.

We are also aware of the creativity and commitment of so many people working in this field and would not want to end this book on a totally pessimistic note. What we consider most important is the openness and authenticity we can glimpse through the self-awareness and reflective practice which years of involvement at the 'sharp end' of mental health practice can bring. Fundamentally we need to foster a willingness to enter into other people's worlds and accept who they are, even if we do not understand all the 'whys'. At the very basic starting point of conscious experience is our individual identity.

10 Additional information

'Human beings ask questions. Our success as a species is due, in no small part, to our quest for knowledge. Underlying a great deal of both what we ask and how we formulate our queries has been our attempt to arrive at an increasingly adequate understanding of ourselves.' (Spinelli 1994)

Key themes:

- Overview
- Myths and MHP
- Definitions

Overview

This last chapter provides the reader with some additional and supporting material. Because the subject of mental health promotion is so broad based, especially in the spectrum of health and social care needs considered, we were not able to include all the relevant information in the chapters as there was so much we would wish to highlight.

Students or those on training courses require useful handouts to take back to workplace/educational settings and to be able to pass on information and ideas. We have provided two pages of definitions/extracts which could be used as discussion points if reproduced. We have also included a glossary of some of the main concepts addressed in Chapter 5 as a focus of discussion. We are aware that there will obviously be other definitions we have not included which might be equally useful or relevant.

In highlighting a few local examples of 'good practice' we are acutely aware of how difficult it is to identify other relevant agencies, and it will be up to the reader to find out what is happening in their locality and perhaps try to disseminate ideas of what constitutes primary, secondary, and tertiary approaches and how MHP should span this.

We have included an outline of the development of the mental health promotion group in our locality and hope that it could also focus discussion or comparisons with other initiatives taking place throughout the country. Part of the work undertaken by Monach and Spriggs is also reproduced in terms of the findings of their small-scale research, as we consider that primary community health care is such an important area, in terms of both practice initiatives and future research and development.

Material identified as relating to each relevant chapter has also been included. This section is essentially an update to enhance existing material. We have also provided more questions to consider and one exercise around mental health promotion that we have found useful in both educational and practice settings. We have listed some useful addresses and further reading, and acknowledge that this list is incomplete.

Finally, we had hoped to undertake research into the educational needs of mental health workers and students regarding mental health promotion, and this has been and will continue to be a primary concern in encouraging reflection and action. We are interested to know how mental health promotion is being taught on health and social care courses. Research is currently being planned and will be evaluated in a further edition of this book.

Above all we hope that our identification of what constitutes mental health promotion, and its relevance to any current debates about the future role of mental health practitioners, is further supported by the approach we have taken. We would wish to encourage others to be interested in and involved in promoting the mental health of us all, as we have been doing and will continue to do.

Chapter 1

In Chapter 1 we set the scene for our identification of what constituted mental health promotion, and our rationale for developing our ideas as we have done. We provide a further focus for discussion in terms of the following.

Myths and MHP

A range of statements and preconceptions may hinder you in taking forward some of the theory and practice we have discussed in the previous chapters. We provide some of these 'myths' and possible responses to enable a clearer dialogue and foundation for practice.

Myth no. 1: 'It's too large a subject'

This argument assumes that factors influencing mental health are so numerous and complex that the task is best left alone. In response we would argue there is a range of low-tech means to support and sustain mental health at the individual and community level. These can have an incremental effect on wider social policy and decisions that affect populations. Empowerment implies change on a subtle and grander scale.

Myth no. 2: 'It's too theoretical'

It can be a philosophical tangle attempting to define and realize what mental health is or is not. Pragmatically we are calling for practitioners to think before they act, drawing on community and user-led solutions to mental health and illness. A social model of mental health is the way forward for practice.

Myth no. 3: 'Solutions and interventions suggested are beyond the scope of health care'

Many of the structural changes and inequalities which affect the potential for good mental health or inhibit recovery from mental illness are broad and can appear distant from day-to-day practice. However, an emphasis on interagency working is seen as central to good practice. Forming and sustaining relationships with housing, social and welfare agencies can contribute to a culture and practice which highlights the determinants of health and does something positively about them.

Myth no. 4: 'We do it anyway'

This is the 'MHP by default' argument. Good practice equals a health-promoting practitioner. We would argue that some practice, however well intentioned, can disempower individuals, groups and communities. Solutions imposed upon groups and populations can reinforce a sense of powerlessness. To examine issues such as oppression and inequality and to practise within a health for all philosophy requires a critical review of current practice.

Myth no. 5: 'It costs too much'

Involvement in MHP practice does have a cost in financial terms and in terms of the capacity for agencies and communities to release staff and resources. The release of imagination, innovation and partnership, on the other hand, is very cost-effective. MHP should not be seen as actively planned and undertaken in isolation. Indeed, you may be a small but significant character in a larger production. Collaborative work has valuable outcomes such as better communication, clarification of roles and responsibilities and improved information. Thinking laterally to consider associated programmes and projects which have a mental health element to them, such as urban and rural regeneration, is a valuable way of achieving a lot for little investment.

Myth no. 6: 'We cannot evaluate it'

Evidence-based practice in nursing and social work has a high profile. MHP in all its guises should be no different. Whether as part of economic regeneration or as a separate piece of work with individuals or groups, attempts to evaluate effectiveness are necessary. The Health Promotion Authority in Wales has funded research testing the effectiveness of mental health projects and identifies 40 that come under the umbrella of prevention, education and MHP. The Health Education Authority is currently developing outcome indicators for MHP and there is a long tradition of community development evaluation.

Myth no. 7: 'We don't have the skills'

MHP is seen as a technical activity requiring resources and training beyond the realm of ordinary practice, or as rooted in community and social models of health far removed from professional practice. There are considerable attitudinal shifts that can and should be built into training and professional practice update. We are all potential users of mental health services and we all operate in the social sphere. As such we have understanding and misunderstanding to formulate emotionally health-enhancing practice. By being exposed and prepared to learn from community work, primary care, and the self-help and user movements, we can become more sophisticated professionals and practitioners of MHP.

Myth no. 8: 'We do not have the time'

The changes in health and social care have placed extra demands upon the statutory, voluntary and independent services. Practice is dynamic and, despite constraints, research, pilot projects, support to other initiatives and general awareness of innovation remain. Joint ventures and a supportive or consultive role are ways in which you can become involved without open-ended commitments. It may be easier to key in to existing initiatives rather than to establish – and reinvent – new ones.

Myth no. 9: 'There is little that can be achieved immediately'

Good communication skills and listening and acting within a public health perspective are deemed essential for the health and social care professions as we move to the next millennium. It is what policy makers, professional bodies and the public want. How practice is implemented, as well as what is practiced, is important. A leaflet or a small project will not radically alter perceptions or society. Yet if the small scale is planned and evaluated and then championed, it can start to sway and influence organizations and the public they serve.

Myth no. 10: 'Our focus is on those with severe and enduring mental illness'

Fear of a practice drift towards people with less disabling mental illness is a concern. We would stress time and again that the principles and philosophy of MHP are based upon the need for the foundations for health to be in place. People with severe and enduring mental illness have as much right for their mental health to be promoted as any citizen. Ensuring access to treatment and care offering choice, control and dignity in partnership with others is a practical step towards promoting the mental health of the mentally ill. Social needs should be met, but there is also a part to play in developing and enhancing the social sphere in which such needs are expressed and satisfied.

The work of Whitehead *et al.* (1995) (see Table 10.1) as outlined in Chapter 1 highlights different levels at which inequalities can be tackled. These levels have a resonance for MHP. Where the practitioner is located – manager, commissioner, clinician, user or carer – may suggest where their energies are best directed. *Where would you place yourself?*

Table 10.1 **Macro, intermediate and micro level interventions for tackling inequalities in health (from Benzeval *et al.* 1995)**	**Macro level**	**Intermediate level**	**Micro level**
	Encourage national and international socioeconomic, cultural and environmental change to enhance health	Create changes in organizations and policies, activities and services to promote health and increase access to essential services and facilities, and to strengthen, support and empower communities	Strengthen, support and empower individuals

The following definitions are intended to provide a focus for discussion in terms of trying to define what we are talking about.

Mental health/psychiatry/mental illness

There is some overlap of terminology in the field of mental state issues. Generally, the differentiation between mental health and mental illness mirrors the way in which we determine what constitutes health and illness across the board. Do we view this as a spectrum, or consider that once illness is classified we are talking about another continuum?

Psychiatry: A branch of medicine that deals with 'diseases' of the mind. Treats classified illness as determined by diagnostic categorization such as ICD 10 and DSM IV. There is still a great deal of confusion and difficulty in assessing whether we are talking about problems with living or stress/distress, or the language problems people have in trying to define how they 'feel', and subsequently behave, in terms of inner and outer sources of conflict. People say they feel depressed or out of control, or are having a 'nervous breakdown'. Is this mental illness? Should front-line treatment primarily reside in the medical domain, however much psychiatrists acknowledge the efficacy of psychopharmacology as being a 'double-edged' sword?

Mental illness: Linked to psychiatry and classification systems, but perhaps more the province of health and social care workers, and spanning primary, secondary and tertiary provision and approaches to this 'problem'. Mental illness is recognized and treated in a variety of ways, but has acute links to legal and statutory requirements of a given society. It helps people to give a 'name' to what they are experiencing, but throws up as many dilemmas as it attempts to solve and has to be viewed in a cultural, political and socioeconomic context.

Mental health: Considered to be a 'desirable' state. Equates to our understanding of emotional well-being, subjectivity, and the attainment of individual potential. Considered in terms of 'self' in the philosophical sense, as in the pursuit of happiness or authenticity, but also realized in strategies to promote it at community and societal levels: 'perhaps mental health and social justice are two sides of the same coin' (Monach and Spriggs 1995).

Mental health promotion: Mental health promotion is the 'action' element of any comprehensive interpretation of everyone's mental health needs and wants. It is underpinned by an anti-oppressive framework for practice which emphasizes cooperative social participation. This is fundamental in realistically addressing the conflictual nature of relationships between the public, professionals and the state.

Chapter 2

In Chapter 2 we examined policy and its impact on mental illness and its relevance for MHP. Some further background information is provided here. Boxes 10.1 and 10.2 summarize recent developments in mental health policy and the ten-point plan for mental health.

Key aspects and issues derived from policy include:

- Empowerment and user-led initiatives
- The advocacy movement
- The changing role and development of mental health workers
- Self-help and the voluntary sector
- A social model of health
- Healthy cities and healthy institutions – public health policy

Box 10.1 **Recent mental health policy developments and government guidance and advice**

1988	Community Care: Agenda for Action. Sir Roy Griffiths
1990	Caring for People. Community Care in the Next Decade and Beyond White Paper NHS and Community Care Act
	House of Commons Social Services Committee Report on Community Care: Services for People with a Mental Handicap and People with a Mental Illness. Community Care in the next Decade and Beyond: Policy Guidance DOH Care Programme Approach.
	Mental Illness Specific Grant
1992	Mental Illness Key Area in Health of the Nation. DOH White Paper
1993	Public Health: Responsibilities of the NHS and the Role of Others. HSG (93)
Aug. 1993	DOH review 'Legal powers on the care of mentally ill people in the community'
Jan. 1994	DOH 'Guidance on the discharge of mentally disordered people from hospital and their continuing care in the community'
Feb. 1994	'Introduction of supervision registers for mentally ill people from April 1 1994.' HSG (94) 5
May 1994	'Guidance on the discharge of mentally disordered people and their continuing care in the community'. HSG (94)
1994	Developing NHS Purchasing and GP Fundholding. Towards a Primary Care-led Service. EL (94) 79
1995	Clinical Standards Advisory Group report on Schizophrenia and request for local reviews

1996	*Building Bridges*: a guide to arrangements for interagency working for the care and protection of severely mentally ill people

Box 10.2 **The mental health ten-point plan (1993, in DOH 1995d)**

1. Powers to supervise the care of patients detained under the 1983 Mental Health Act requiring special support after hospital discharge
2. Publication of the DOH report of its review of the 1983 Mental Health Act
3. Publication of a new version of the code of practice
4. Guidance on the discharge of psychiatric patients from hospital
5. Better training for key workers in their duties under the Care Programme Approach
6. Development of better information systems and a special supervision register of patients who may be at risk and need most support
7. A review by the Clinical Standards Advisory Group of standards of care for people with schizophrenia
8. A work programme for the Mental Health Task Force to support health authorities moving to locally based care
9. Ensuring that the health authority and GP fundholder purchasing plans cover the essential needs for mental health services
10. An action programme to help improve mental health services in London

The Care Programme Approach

The Care Programme Approach (CPA) was introduced in 1991 to provide a framework for the care of the mentally ill outside of hospital settings. This will obviously be dependent on the requirements of a particular locality in terms of the financial investment afforded to individuals, but will be more concerned to clarify assessment in terms of risk and dangerousness. There are four key parts to it:

1. An assessment of health and social care needs
2. A plan of care
3. Nomination of a key worker to coordinate care
4. A regular review of circumstances.

Assessment

This seeks to identify health and social needs. This can be as limiting or boundless as desired. The work of Leader (1995) and others in this field shows the possibilities for expanding assessment into an empowering tool in its own right, highlighting strengths as much as weaknesses for the user and carer involved in the process.

A plan of care

The product of an assessment process should be a plan of care and support that responds to the needs and wants expressed as part of the assessment. A major difficulty has been in matching wants, needs and limited resources. This is where the importance of a raft of specialist and nonspecialist support is evident.

Key workers

The identification of a named key worker or care coordinator is a vital element in the CPA. It should ensure a continuity and a responsibility by the statutory agency to fulfil its duty in terms of pulling together all the disparate parts which make up and sustain a range of care for the client concerned.

Review

Another function of the coordinating role is to ensure that there is an adequate review of changes in circumstances of individuals and of the services that provide care and support. Much of the contemporary literature such as the Mental Health Act Commission (1995) emphasize the importance of user and care involvement in all aspects of the CPA process, but particularly of systematic review to identify gaps and changed care needs. A significant issue for MHP is the role of the person experiencing the CPA. The Mental Health Foundation Report (1994) makes a series of conclusions and recommendations to commissioning authorities. These include recommendations that people who use mental health service provision should be directly involved in service development and evaluation and that there should be a use of independent advocates. Recommendations 37 and 38 are to:

- Establish panels of service users to advise on the development and evaluation of services for people with severe mental illness
- Ensure that people on supervision registers are offered the assistance of a suitable advocate

Such recommendations have been echoed by MIND in its Policy on Community Care (1995) and its 'BreakThrough' campaign aimed at making community care work (1994c). These have been responses to the reality of users and carers experiencing the new government mental health policy in action. They call for national minimum standards for quality community care, access to crisis services and wider choice and information on services and medications.

Public health nursing role and implications for sets of the nursing profession

The policy shift towards primary and community-focused practice for nursing is extending all the time. Table 10.2 identifies the key elements of future practice.

Nursing area	Recommendation/focus
District nursing	Clinical audit, guidelines and protocols for practice
General practice nursing	Population approaches to primary prevention and a social context of health
Health visitor nursing	Health promotion/prevention activity specified and research outcomes of work in areas of poverty/nonpoverty
Learning disability/mental health nursing	Community participation – involvement of local communities in planning of services
Midwifery nursing	Primary preventive education, client participation and needs assessment
Occupational health nursing	Men's health and workplace policy development
School nursing	Assessing effectiveness of interventions and adoption of a population approach
Secondary care nursing	Hospital-based health promotion and enhancing dialogue with primary care
Specialist nursing	Vehicle to link a health-promoting hospital with community-orientated primary care
Practice nursing	Identifying preventive approaches in a social context of health

Table 10.2
Key elements for future nursing practice

Chapter 3

In Chapter 3 we examined community participation and health alliances as a vehicle for promoting mental health. There is plenty of opportunity for the practitioner to become involved in such activity and we include further details of examples discussed.

Wallace (1993) examined local social networks and highlighted certain conditions which in combination enable communities experiencing poverty and deprivation to improve health. Essentially, using community development as a strategy, thriving and dynamic communities – urban and rural – can enhance social cohesion and promote overall perceptions and experiences to promote health (see Box 10.3).

Box 10.3 **Creating healthier conditions for a poor community**

- Social control of illegal activity and substance misuse
- Socialization of the young as participating members of a community
- Limiting the duration and intensity of youthful experimentation with dangerous and destructive activity
- Providing first employment
- Improving access to formal and informal health care
- Social support for maintaining health
- Political power to direct resources and deflect threats

(Wallace 1993)

Healthy Sheffield's Framework for Action (1994)

Box 10.4 presents the Framework for Action.

Box 10.4 **Healthy Sheffield's Framework for Action**

Section 2 FRAMEWORK FOR ACTION
H. Mental & Emotional Well-being

IMPORTANCE TO HEALTH
Emotional well-being is one of the bases of good physical and mental health.

Stress and emotional problems undermine people's quality of life and can cause physical ill-health.

Mental illness is distressing for sufferers and their families and friends.

Emotional problems can drive people to substance misuse, self-harm and suicide.

PROBLEMS FOR PARTICULAR GROUPS

Women can feel isolated and under pressure from their role as carers, their dual burden of work and care, the absence of child care and social support and as a result of their position in society, women from some minority ethnic communities are particularly vulnerable to isolation.

Men are often unwilling to acknowledge stress and emotional problems, which can lead to stress-related and mental ill-health.

Lesbians and gay men can experience abuse, harassment and racist violence which undermine their emotional, as well as physical health.

Children and young people can experience low self-esteem particularly if they are not cared for or are abused. Lack of support and affection through the process of growing up can cause severe stress and emotional problems.

Older people are vulnerable to isolation and loneliness and need social support to cope with some of the problems of growing older in our society.

Unemployed people, particularly the long-term unemployed, experience low self-esteem, isolation and poverty.

People in poverty are under acute emotional pressure from having to make ends meet and because of poor access to health-promoting activities.

People with mental illness need adequate support to live in the community with as much independence as possible.

WHAT SHOULD WE BE TRYING TO ACHIEVE?

1. The reduction of sources of stress, targeted towards the most vulnerable groups
2. The provision of appropriate support for people mentally ill or under stress
3. The promotion of emotional well-being through the provision of opportunities for self and community development.

AREAS FOR ACTION

1. Reducing Stress

Research and information on the contributory factors to poor mental health in specific groups.

Enabling local communities and groups to define their own needs for social support.

Community projects aimed at reducing social isolation and establishing support networks for key groups.

Provision of child care, carers' support initiatives and family support.

Interagency action to promote self-esteem for all children and young people, particularly those abused and neglected.

2. Providing Support

Extension of community mental health services.

Improving the accessibility of counselling and psychotherapeutic services, particularly to black and minority ethnic people.

Group-based therapy and discussion, targeted towards socially isolated groups and communities.

Support services for victims of crime, harassment and abuse.

Information and training for health and other service professionals to identify emotional problems and provide appropriate support.

Support for voluntary sector organizations which provide self-help, networking and advocacy for people suffering stress and isolation.

Extending the range of accommodation with support and care for people with mental health problems.

3. Promotion

Development of projects to promote good mental health.

Provision of opportunities for social contact targeted at key groups.

Employment and training opportunities for key groups.

Activities for children and young people which enable them to develop social and emotional skills.

Education on healthy relationships.

Strategies for community participation and involvement in planning and decision-making.

CROSS-REFERENCES
Sexual Health & Fertility,
Work, Smoking, Alcohol & Drugs,
Discrimination, Violence & Aggression,
Poverty

Healthy Alliances

An example of education and youth service activity is given in Table 10.3.

Table 10.3 **MHP targets, interventions and outcomes in a school setting**	Health of the Nation targets (G. McCulloch, unpublished data)	Possible interventions	Outcomes
	Reduce the incidence of mental illness and suicide	Develop school counselling initiatives	Reduction in stress and suicide
(continued opposite)	Demystify mental illness and raise public awareness of positive mental health	Implement mental health education within curriculum	Increased knowledge of mental health and mental illness

Health of the Nation targets (G. McCulloch, unpublished data)	Possible interventions	Outcomes	Table 10.3 **MHP targets, interventions and outcomes in a school setting** *(continued)*
Prevent the deterioration of an existing mental illness	Early detection and referral mechanisms including policy	Improved quality and appropriateness of referrals	
Improve the quality of life for people with mental health problems	Establish close links between adult education and community mental health agencies	Development of new skills and training opportunities out of clinical environment	
Maintain and improve social functioning	Self-esteem and social skills	Participants develop and utilize new skills	

Chapter 4

In Chapter 4 we described strategic approaches to MHP. In the Sheffield context as part of the Sheffield Strategy for Adult Mental Health (1996) the following approach has been agreed.

Promoting mental and emotional well-being

Factors affecting mental health

Many factors can influence the onset of mental illness and have a significant impact on the degree, severity and longer-term damage caused by mental ill-health. Work to promote mental and emotional well-being should address a range of factors, including:

- Physiological factors
- Housing
- Community support
- Social relationships and friendship networks
- Family and carer support
- Employment
- Recreation

Objectives

The statutory agencies will need to pursue the following objectives, partly through their own direct work and partly by influencing the activities of others in the community:

- To build healthy communities, ensuring a multiagency approach to the problems faced by many communities in Sheffield
- To build community support infrastructures
- To develop comprehensive public education programmes, adapted to the needs of particular communities, to challenge the stigma attached to mental illness and to raise public awareness
- To extend the multiagency response to carers' needs and support for carers' services
- To encourage user and community participation in assessing needs and identifying gaps in service provision

A Healthy Alliance approach

Within the framework of Healthy Sheffield, the agencies should work to build alliances with other organizations to influence the many factors which affect individuals' and communities' mental health and well-being.

Support for carers and communities

The agencies should support and contribute to community activities which seek to empower people. A community development approach should be encouraged to develop supportive community infrastructures and informal support networks.

All work around adult mental health should be aimed at assisting individuals within the context of their own networks of carers, families and friends and at supporting those networks.

Countering difference

Stigma and discrimination are strongly associated with mental illness. The agencies should develop regular public education initiatives designed to improve understanding of the issues. These should be adapted to the needs of particular communities, including black and minority ethnic communities, and should involve schools and community groups.

The agencies are already committed to equality of opportunity and to challenging prejudice and oppression. Part of implementing this should be to consider how they themselves as organizations influence mental health and the development of policies and practice in ways which support the mental health of employees and others.

Interagency training and education

Work to promote positive approaches to mental health should include an increased emphasis on joint training and education initiatives for staff. Agencies should develop and integrate into their training pro-grammes a variety of training opportunities around mental health issues. The skills and experiences of partner agencies should increasingly be shared as part of this process.

Information and research

The agencies should encourage user, carer and wider community participation in assessing needs and identifying gaps in mental health provision.

Chapter 5

In our discussion of education and training we highlighted the dilemmas of practice and also some possible solutions. Below are two examples.

How to promote mental health in an acute setting

- **Acknowledge that it is possible:** People with an acute mental illness still have mental and emotional well-being capacity, needs and resources. This needs to be accepted and worked on. Mental health and its promotion must be part of assessment, treatment and rehabilitation.
- **Accept strengths, abilities and capabilities:** Recognize and be sympathetic to cultural, religious and other needs. Ensure that spiritual as well as social and medical needs are met.
- **Respect solutions and strategies that the person in your care has for dealing with their distress:** Try to incorporate them in any plan of care, however trivial they may seem.
- **Ask 'normal' questions about people:** Ask how they are – as much for the human nature of it as for assessing and monitoring changes in symptoms and condition. Be clear and honest with people when the questioning is part of a formal assessment process.
- **Use the contact you have wisely:** Have openness about your role in the recording and monitoring of conditions. Clarify where this ends and where genuine social contact begins. Maintain information and contact with a broad range of helping agencies and services beyond the hospital.
- **Accept that a psychiatric inpatient facility is not a 'normal' place either in design or purpose:** It is to offer assessment, treatment, safety, sanctuary and security and is temporary. As such it is not a home, and all efforts should be made to link with supported and other forms of housing from day one.

- **Be clear about current policy on discrimination:** Ensure that everyone is aware of this and monitor its impact.
- **Identify how the clinical environment can be made more relevant to the needs of users and carers:** Exploit a range of information, contacts, calendars, benefits advice, advocacy and self-help as well as key agencies.

A training exercise for discussion of MHP

To stimulate debate on what MHP is and how we can initiate action in this area we have used an exercise with students centred around the following tasks.

(A) Split into two groups and, using a range of media, try to imagine an 'ideal' mentally healthy town or city. What would it consist of? What would it require to achieve and maintain the status of a mentally healthy environment? What are the possible threats?

The results are shared and discussed and emerging themes are logged.

(B) This is followed by a second task which involves two groups each with a separate task. Following from the previous 'brainstorming' of an ideal community, the groups are asked to plan a range of actions and interventions which they can justify as being able to promote the mental health of a population. (This can be refined to focus on a particular area or community.) The first group is provided with significant resources to do this – a grant of one million pounds to develop MHP. The second group is asked to complete the same task within existing resources.

Tools to assist them include a range of documents, papers and resources such as health promotion theory and models, local and national health and social policy documents, examples of health alliances, mental health strategies, prevention and educational literature, purchasing plans, good practice from the user and self-help movement, particularly from oppressed and marginalized groups.

The results are then shared and differences and similarities in approach are considered. Key aspects to identify: Have mental illness as well as mental health needs been identified? How far have the resources been used to inform decision making? How has decision making been shaped and influenced by preconceived ideas about race, culture, gender, sexuality, social class and community?

The exercise can also be refined to consist of a 'competition' between the two groups to formulate a plan to spend one million pounds.

Glossary

This glossary is intended to support the issues that are raised throughout the book but are considered more relevant to Chapter 5, although the issues are also raised in Chapters 1 and 9. These definitions could also be used for discussion.

Accountability   Liability; being answerable for one's own actions; the need to explain and justify decisions taken or activities performed, as the best course available within prevailing circumstances. Accountability is awarded in an authority to act, and requires detailed knowledge of the proposed course of action, the alternatives available, the potential implications and repercussions of each, to be weighed in reaching a conclusion. (Thompson and Mathias 1994, *Mental Health and Disorder*, p. 657)

Advocacy   Based on the notion of enabling users to articulate their needs and ensuring that their rights are respected. When users are unable to speak up for themselves and do not have the capacity to decide what type of needs they have or how they would like them to be met, then the advocate will have to act in what is judged to be their best interests. (Banks 1995, *Ethics and Values in Social Work*, p. 111)

Anti-oppressive practice   . . . minimizing the power differences in society. Such practice 'works with a model of empowerment and liberation and requires as fundamental rethinking of values, institutions and relationships'. (Phillipson 1992, in Dalrymple and Burke 1995, *Anti-Oppressive Practice: Social Care and the Law*, p. 3)

Antiracist practice   An antiracist perspective focuses on transforming the unequal social relations shaping social interaction between black and white people into egalitarian ones . . . . What both black and antiracist perspectives have in common is a commitment to social change in order to eradicate racism. (Dominelli 1997b, *Anti Racist Social Work*, 2nd edn., p. 33)

Assessment   Assessment and analysis of assessment data involves sifting through information to identify and understand patterns, interrelationships and meanings assigned to various aspects of the data. Whether or not it is consciously acknowledged, we continually analyse or assign meaning to information. The meanings assigned are shaped by past experiences, cultural orientations, professional expectations, and a variety of other influences of which we may be only partially aware. It must be kept in mind that assessment and interpretation are never totally objective. They help create and shape the facts, innuendoes and inferences that are important to the application of the problem-solving process. (Kavanagh and Kennedy 1992, *Promoting Cultural Diversity*, p. 102)

Autonomy   Autonomy (literally, self-rule) is, in summary, the capacity to think, decide, and act on the basis of such thought and decision freely and independently . . . . Autonomy is sometimes subdivided into autonomy of action, autonomy of will and autonomy of thought . . . . In the sphere of action it is important to distinguish between, on the one hand, freedom, liberty, licence, or simply doing what one wants to do and, on the other hand, acting autonomously, which may also be doing what one wants to do but on the basis of thought or reasoning. (Gillon 1985, *Philosophical Medical Ethics*, p. 60)

Black   We follow Bandana Ahmad's (1990) terminology in use of the word 'black', which is used to describe people mainly from South Asian, African, and Caribbean backgrounds and other visible minorities in Britain. We do not use the term 'black' to deny difference and diversity. The term 'black' is used in a political sense to reflect the struggles of nonwhite groups against the oppression they experience from white institutions. The expression of being 'black' is a source of unified strength and solidarity. (Dalrymple and Burke, *op. cit.*; p. xv)

Caring   As an ongoing process, care consists of four analytically separate, but interconnected phases. They are: caring about, taking care of, care-giving and care-receiving . . . . Care is perhaps best thought of as a practice. The notion of a practice is complex; it is an alternative to conceiving of care as a principle or an emotion. (Tronto 1993, *Moral Boundaries: A Political Argument for an Ethics of Care*, p. 105)

Community work   Community work is frequently seen as providing a radical alternative to other forms of social intervention, an opportunity to tackle causes rather than bandage systems. In fact, community work like social work is open to a variety of ideological perspectives; from conservative strategies for social control or schemes to off-load statutory responsibilities onto deprived communities, through technocratic attempts to define a more sophisticated skill base for community work, to various strands of radicalism. (Craig, Derricourt and Loney 1982, *Community Work and the State*, p. 1)

Community   Community, then, is a term to be wary of since it lacks a coherent definition, at least in current usage. Under present conditions, it has been successfully co-opted by the dominant ideology and has become another facet of possessive individualism. In cases where the term is used to denote some sort of collectivist or socialized approach to issues of responsibility, it is better for the sake of clarity to stick with those terms themselves. The continued use of the word 'community' simply obfuscates it. (Dalley 1996, *Ideologies of Caring: Rethinking Community and Collectivism*, p. 56)

Critical education   We are strongly motivated to work towards critical education in the belief that it is empowering education. We believe that education should involve students in efforts to identify their own problems, to critically analyse the historical, cultural and socio-economic roots of these and to develop strategies to create positive change in their lives and communities. (Green, Martin and Williams 1996, Critical Consciousness or Commercial Consciousness; in Humphries 1996, *Critical Perspectives on Empowerment*, p. 117)

Culture An identity which everyone has, based on a number of factors, such as: memories, ethnic identity, family attitudes to child-rearing, class, money, religious or other celebrations, division of family roles according to gender and age. Cultures are neither superior nor inferior to each other. They are constantly evolving for individuals and communities. (Macdonald 1991, *All Equal Under the Act: A Practice Guide to the Children's Act*)

Dialectic Art/practice of assessing the truth of a theory by discussion and logical disputation – interpretive method – contradictions resolved at a higher level of truth (synthesis). (*New Collins Dictionary*)

Disabled Having a physical, emotional or learning impediment requiring the provision of specific facilities to enable the individual to participate in, contribute to, and benefit from, both their personal life and the full rights and responsibilities of citizenship, insofar as they choose to do so. (Macdonald, *op. cit.*; p. xx)

Eurocentric Looking at, exclusively valuing and interpreting the world through the eyes and experiences of white Europeans. This includes, for example, the presentation and interpretation of historical events; defining of 'correct' methods of child rearing and organizing family life; seeing Europe as the centre of the world. (Macdonald, *op. cit.*; p. xx)

Empowerment Empowerment, particularly in health and social literature, is usually understood to mean 'to give a voice to, to enable, and developing individuals' ability to help themselves'. It is variously described as being about citizenship, rights, responsibilities and needs. Expressed in terms of 'having a say', user involvement, exercising power and control, taking charge and sometimes in terms of changing society but more usually it is about changing the individual. (Carabine 1996, in Humphries 1996, *Critical Perspectives on Empowerment*, p. 30)

Ethnicity Refers to individuals' identification with a group sharing some or all of the following traits: customs, lifestyles, religion, language, nationality. In the context of this society, the 'racial factor' influences individuals' definition of their own ethnicity (such as black/Asian, black/Caribbean). It is important to remember that white people also belong to ethnic groups. (Macdonald, *op. cit.*; p. xx)

Homophobia Discrimination based on heterosexual beliefs. Both personal and institutional, it is supported by legislation affecting family life, employment, immigration rights and civil liberties. (Macdonald, *op. cit.*; p. xx)

Ideology A useful concept which helps analyse the interrelations of conflict and consensus is that of *ideology* – values and beliefs which help secure the position of more powerful groups at the expense of less powerful ones. Power, ideology and conflict are always closely connected. Many conflicts are *about* power, because of the rewards it can bring. Those who hold most power may depend mainly on the influences of ideology to retain their dominance, but they are usually able also to use force if necessary. (Giddens 1993, *Sociology*, 2nd edn., p. 722)

Minority ethnic   Belonging to a cultural, racial or religious group that is numerically smaller than the predominantly white protestant majority power base in the United Kingdom. This includes groups visible on the basis of their skin colour, as well as such as Irish, Jewish, Polish, Turkish and Travelling peoples. Belonging can come either through personal identification with a group through the allocation by others or individuals to it. (Macdonald, *op. cit.*; p. xx)

Need   MIND – in line with the disabled living movement – believes that the right and opportunity to live independently and equally with others is the starting point for a user-centred approach to needs assessment. (MIND 1995, *Reshaping the Future: MIND's Model for Community Mental Health Care*)

Oppression   The word oppress comes from the Latin *opprimere*, which means to press on, or to press against. It has been defined as 'Inhuman or degrading treatment of individuals or groups; hardship and injustice brought about by the dominance of one group over another; the negative and demeaning exercise of power. Oppression often involves disregarding the rights of an individual or group and is thus the denial of citizenship'. (Thompson 1995:31, in Dalrymple and Burke, *op. cit.*; p. xvi)

Racism   Racism is therefore, a socially created phenomenon which structures social interaction between black and white people in inegalitarian ways. Racism operates at three levels: the personal, institutional and cultural . . . . Each one of them contributes to the maintenance and reproduction of the others. Hence, to successfully dismantle racism, we need to address all three of these levels, preferably simultaneously. However, this is difficult for one individual to undertake all on his or her own. Hence it is important to form alliances with others inside the workplace and in the broader society – amongst people and organizations who share a commitment to developing a nonoppressive world. (Dominelli, *op. cit.*; p. 23)

Reflective practitioner   By a competent reflective practitioner, I mean someone who: has the knowledge and skills to 'do the job'; can draw on theoretical perspectives to contextualize what they are doing, that is, place it in its socioeconomic and political context; can evaluate their interventions; and can reflect critically upon their own and others' work. (Dominelli, *op. cit.*; p. 33)

Social care   This term is used to describe the activities and processes undertaken by all sectors or agencies, statutory, voluntary and independent, which seek to enable individuals, families and groups who are disadvantaged or deprived in some way to achieve a higher, self-determined level of functioning and quality of life. It is about the planned meeting of client's needs. It concerns the physical, intellectual, emotional, cultural and social aspects of the client's development and well-being. It involves mutual trust and respect; it involves a sense of purpose and change; it recognizes the interaction between people and their environments. (Mallison 1998:1, in Dalrymple and Burke, *op. cit.*; p. xxiii)

Want   As defined by service users' draws attention to ordinary human experience rather than medical labels and may be more conducive to developing a user-centred assessment process. It deals with what is useful to every individual and enables people to match up their aspirations and ambitions with their care plan and the service on offer. The possibility for achievement encourages greater self-esteem and self-empowerment, and allows ordinary local resources to be brought into consideration as ways of improving quality of life for users. Above all, a user-centred assessment process increases informed consent and choice, by providing users with a greater say in decision-making. (MIND, *op. cit.*)

Chapter 6

In Chapter 6 we looked at prevention and education and the strengths and weaknesses of such approaches. It was evident that unless they are part and parcel of a community development model, healthy public policy and partnership working, they will fail. Two templates are provided to show how a preventive and educative approach to Health of the Nation can be considered from the Mental Illness Key Area and more broadly the second includes a range of health issues and possible MHP interventions with a preventive/educational focus.

Health of the Nation targets

Table 10.4 is a template for development of an action plan using Health of the Nation Targets and suggested action using education and youth services. This could be done at a local or a strategic level:

Table 10.4 **Education and youth services (example in italics)**	**Targets**	**Action plan**
	Reduce the incidence of mental illness and suicide	*Develop school counselling initiative. Develop support for young carers and youth services, school nursing services to offer a range of emotional health activity*
	Demystify mental illness and raise public awareness of positive mental health	*Mental health education as part of the curriculum (personal and social education) and in youth service provision*
	Prevent the deterioration of an existing mental illness	*Early detection and appropriate referral to specialist services – develop guidelines and systems for referral*
	Improve the quality of life for people with mental health problems	*Closer liaison between adult education and training agencies' services and community mental health agencies*
	Maintain and improve social functioning	*Establish specific programmes on coping, social skills and assertiveness*

Table 10.5 highlights the relevance of mental health to a wide array of work areas for mental health practitioners and also emphasizes the need to operate at the individual and community–social level.

Table 10.5 **Areas of relevance for mental health and MHP**	**Health issue**	**Mental health aspect**	**MHP intervention**
	Women's health	Domestic violence	Self-help and improvements in service recognition of the problem
	Smoking	Coping and stress	Individual and group methods and skills to minimize stress
	Workplace health	Stress	Individual programmes and some organizational development
	Primary health care	Stress/anxiety	Detection and management of stress, anxiety and depression. Guidelines, protocols and training

(continued opposite)

Health issue	Mental health aspect	MHP intervention	
Substance misuse	Prevention	A range of education strategies in school, youth and other settings	Table 10.5 **Areas of relevance for mental health and MHP** (*continued*)
Child health	Child care/parent support	Individual and group training and skill enhancement in relation to parenting and coping	
Young people	Anti-bullying	Training and education in schools. Policy development	
Sexual health	Self-esteem	Individual and group training and skill acquiring. Anti-oppressive culture	
Coronary heart disease	Stress	Stress relief by tackling the causes of stress – environmental and social	
Accidents	Stress	Education and recognition of effects of stress and accidents	
Older adults	Carers	Loss and adaptation. Social support	
Our own mental health			

Chapter 7

In Chapter 7 we examined the relevance of the NHS reforms to health and social care and suggested ways to positively exploit this to promote mental health. Further background information is provided in Box 10.5.

Box 10.5 **Elements of the purchasing process**

- **Standards and contract specification:** Standard setting is about targets and standards. Standards are part of the process enabling service developments to occur. This is also about setting out the principles for purchasing, for example, Health for All principles
- **Priorities:** A phrase that is increasingly part of the purchasing repertoire and which links in to rationing and redirecting resources. If we could start afresh with health services as well as health problems, the issue of priorities would be relatively straightforward. However, there are

historical patterns of hospital and other service provision. Add to this technological advances and higher expectations of services, and prioritizing purely according to health need becomes more complex

- **Monitoring:** In order to demonstrate the effectiveness or not of service delivery and quality, monitoring of the activity that is provided is required. This is the area in which service users, carers and lobby groups can, potentially, have a considerable influence in the way in which such monitoring takes place
- **Outcomes:** The premise on which the arrangements are based is not to simply replicate traditional patterns of service provision. Rather it is to achieve health gain and improve the quality of service provision. Key outcomes from a service user perspective are improved service developments, increased information, and improved communication and structural changes
- **Audit:** Another phenomenon of the health reforms has been the increase in clinical and organizational audit. This also feeds into the purchasing arena in terms of identifying cost-effective and quality services. The opportunities for the user, carer, voluntary as well as professional input into this should not be underestimated and should be positively sought

Figure 10.1 is a schematic composite of the purchasing process.

Figure 10.1 **The purchasing cycle**

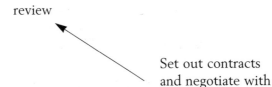

Develop health strategy and policy

Assess health needs

Establish service specifications

Monitor contracts, review

Set out contracts and negotiate with providers

In which parts of this cycle do you consider your practice to be most determined, and why?

The MHP shopping list

Magowan (1994) states that the purchasing 'shopping list' (described in Chapter 7) is intended to highlight key purchasing elements which can be developed into a comprehensive package to promote the mental health of a population. Eight suggested elements which should be present in all NHS contracts are listed in Table 10.6.

Element	
1. The Patients' Charter	Table 10.6 **Elements which should be present in all NHS contracts**
2. An equal opportunities policy	
3. Working in partnership with users to develop services	
4. Encouraging the development of life-skills and self-efficacy	
5. Ensuring access to services by providing information about their availability and promoting what they offer	
6. Support the personal and professional development of staff and patients	
7. Provision of effective communication systems within and between organizations	
8. Provision of health promotion activities based on appropriate health needs assessment.	

Chapter 8

In Chapter 8 we looked at the strength of the user movement and its importance in the field of MHP. At a policy level the background to emerging interest in public participation (see Chapter 3) and user-led services comes in the shape of Local Voices and the Patients' Charter. Further detail is presented here.

Making Local Voices Heard in Purchasing or Health: Annex A (16) in *Local Voices* (NHS Executive 1992)

Assessment of health need	Need to listen: local people will have clear views on needs and relative impact of different services
Purchasing plan	Need to inform local people of purchasing intentions and give a chance to discuss and comment

Service specifications	Need to ensure views expressed are reflected in service specifications
Negotiated contracts	Need to report what these mean and listen to reaction
Contract monitoring	Listen and local people can help in this process
Review of outcomes	Report back to local people on impact of services on health and performance of providers. Listen to views about services

The Patients' Charter

Launched in 1991, the Patients' Charter was aimed at setting out a person's right to NHS care through a set of national standards. It consists of the rights listed in Box 10.6.

Box 10.6 **The Patients' Charter**

The right to receive health care on the basis of clinical needs, regardless of ability to pay

The right to be registered with a GP

The right to be referred to a consultant acceptable to you when your GP thinks it necessary, and to be referred for a second opinion if you and your GP agree this is desirable

The right to have access to your health records

The right to be given a clear explanation of any treatment proposed, including any risks or alternatives, before you decide whether you will agree to the treatment

The guaranteed admission to treatment within two years

The right to have any complaints about NHS services investigated

The right to detailed information on local health services

(DOH 1991)

Chapter 9

In this chapter we considered a small-scale research study undertaken in Sheffield during 1992–3 and the summary contained within it is reproduced here (Box 10.7) to further support our identification of the value of MHP and some of the main challenges it faces.

Box 10.7 **Mental health promotion in Sheffield**

Executive Summary

- The concept of Mental Health Promotion (MHP) is long standing but commands with individual professionals a low level of consensus on its meaning and its relationship to health education and illness prevention. However, semantic debates can obscure the well-established case for interventions which address social and environmental causes and precipitants of mental ill-health as well as those factors linked to relapse and deterioration of those with established mental illness or disorder

- A substantial majority of those interviewed see MHP as a helpful concept

- There is a significant level of professional indifference and even hostility to MHP in part, at least, related to perceptions that treatment and Health Promotion draw on the same budgets, competing for inadequate resources. This concern was particularly evident amongst GPs and psychiatrists

- The reluctance of the psychiatric professions to engage in MHP wholeheartedly is perhaps surprising giving the limited efficacy of many traditional psychiatric interventions

- Despite the reservations amongst some professional groups (notably psychiatrists and doctors), there was strong support for giving MHP some priority – $1/2$ seeing it as essential and $2/5$ as integral to their work

- The range of understandings about MHP found in theoretical writings reviewed in this report was well illustrated by key informants interviewed and questionnaire respondents

- Definitions of MHP which related to community awareness of mental illness were especially popular

- For MHP to develop, the medical profession, particularly psychiatrists, will need convincing of its potential. At present there is a danger that MHP will develop separately as a vehicle for the aspirations of non-medical mental health professionals alone. It is difficult to see that this will benefit the targets of MHP, which should include those with histories of mental ill-health, in the long run

- There was a tendency to view MHP in a primary preventive role exclusively, rather than seeing its potential at secondary and tertiary levels also. It is partly this concentration which raises the scepticism of psychiatric professionals

- Both extremes of HP approach were represented in our research – those advocating community development and others changed lifestyles. Partly because of the political undertones associated with the approaches, consensus is likely to be limited. No single approach is likely to command universal acceptance, although at an agency level Healthy Sheffield policies encourage certain emphases

- There was a disappointing level of knowledge about actual MHP activities or, at least, very restricted definitions of what might be considered MHP

- There was a low level of appreciation of the MHP aspects of the work of core mental health services

- Only 1:4 of mental health professionals surveyed claimed involvement in a MHP activity or project. This was well below the level of knowledge of such activities. Just 5% saw MHP as a significant part of their role

- Only 4% mentioned knowledge of the MHP Project, although their comments were all positive. The MHP Project was seen by this small group as generally very positive and even crucial in the development of over a dozen significant mental health service developments in the City. Health personnel were seen as significantly more committed than others to MHP

- MHP Policies were not generally well known – only about one third of those working in settings with such policies. However, those aware of the policies were overwhelmingly positive about their impact on individual practice

- Women respondents tended in general to have more positive attitudes

- At least $^2/_3$ of all professional groups would give more time to MHP if time and resources allowed

- There was a high level of concern to address issues of perceived widespread poor mental health in the community

- There was little emphasis on MHP in training received, especially amongst psychiatrists, according to respondents. This suggests a need for training amongst those in senior and influential positions

- Interviewees tended to emphasize the key role of primary care in the development of MHP

- Only $^1/_4$ of the respondents felt they had a lead role in MHP. GPs and psychiatrists were least likely to claim this standing. This reinforced for us the concern that these key professionals may be marginalized in this area and MHP be the loser as a result

Further reading

There are so many books relevant to mental health promotion that it is difficult to attempt any comprehensive listing. The books cited as references would be an informative start to this subject.

There are increasingly more books written from the perspective of user involvement and MIND produces regular updates of books available, as well as useful video/training material, such as *Anger to Action*. There is also a wide range of leaflets on mental health promotion and other important subjects, such as the law and mental illness. MIND's current list includes all aspects of mental health and illness and covers a wide range of opinions and debate. We have highlighted some of these and added other relevant titles that we are more familiar with.

A very useful approach to general reading around this subject is to consider the material in the Icon publications – *Psychiatry for Beginners*, *Philosophy for Beginners*, *Medicine for Beginners*, *Feminism for Beginners*, etc. They are not expensive and are useful as a focus for discussion and handouts. The authors use a cartoon format and drawings that are insightful and relevant to 'professionals' and the public alike.

An equally useful approach to training and exercises around mental health/mental illness/mental health promotion is to use the resources available from Pavilion Publishing. If these are not available in local community libraries, they would be in the libraries of health promotion departments and are open to the public as well as health and social care staff. These packs are useful in that they examine issues from a wide range of perspectives and include community care as a central focus. A recent training pack is relevant for those with a learning disability and mental health problems, and identifies the recent interest in 'dual needs'.

For students, learning where to access useful material is an integral part of the educational process and we all know how hard it is either to pay for books or try to grab what is on offer in relevant libraries before someone else does. It is hoped that an important part of therapeutic care would be to provide a learning environment, as well as a clinical one, not only for students but for trained staff and the people they are helping to resolve a wide range of problems. There are many works of fiction that consider the 'felt' experience of mental illness, or how individual 'identity' becomes subsumed within this process. MIND, in their publication list, puts these under the heading of 'grassroots' reading. If there were more material available like this, in clinical areas, for example – not only books but the journals that have mental health as their focus – it might further encourage the initiatives taking place in terms of user-led involvement in mental health provision and practice.

General sources

Grassroots is a bi-monthly newsletter of the Mental Health Task Force produced by the NHS Executive and is intended to keep people in touch on a range of mental health issues. It provides examples of good practice, local initiatives and key policy issues on mental health.

OpenMind is a monthly magazine produced by the national mental health charity, MIND, and provides a range of articles, debate and information on a whole range of mental health news, views and activity.

Other relevant journals include, *Mental Health Nursing, Journal of Psychiatric and Mental Health Nursing, Asylum, Community Care. Nursing Times* provides a useful resource for consideration of all aspects of nursing care and maintains a high profile for mental health issues. *Health Matters* is a journal looking at public health from a more radical perspective, and is published monthly.

Mastering how to surf the 'psychiatric information superhighway', and being aware of the increasing number of relevant CD-Roms is difficult, but is an essential part of the process of developing expertise in information technology, both as a learning strategy, and in helping to identify what is happening at a global level in terms of understanding of our mental health needs and how to promote them.

Men/women/children

Abel K *et al.* (eds), *Planning Community Mental Health Services for Women*. Routledge.
Barnes M and Maple N, *Women and Mental Health: Challenging the Stereotypes*. Venture Press, 1992.
Buningham S, *Young People Under Stress*. MIND/Virago, 1994.
Busfield J, *Men, Women and Madness: Understanding Gender and Mental Disorder*. Macmillan, 1996.
David T (ed.), *Working Together for Young Children*. Routledge, 1994.
Doyal L, *What Makes Women Sick: Gender and the Political Economy of Health*. Macmillan, 1995.
Gorman J, *Out of the Shadows*. MIND, 1992.
Hughes B, *Older People and Community Care*. Open University Press, 1995.
Lago C, *Race, Culture and Counselling*. Open University Press, 1996.
Meth RL and Pasick R, *Men in Therapy: The Challenge of Change*. Guildford Press, 1994.
Slater R, *The Psychology of Growing Old*. Open University Press, 1995.
Spandler H, *Who's Hurting Who? Young People, Self-Harm and Suicide*. 42nd Street, 1996.
Ussher J, *Women's Madness: Misogyny or Mental Illness*. Harvester Wheatsheaf, 1991.
Zaki M and others, *Inside Outside*. Outsider Publications, 1995.

Gender/ethnicity

Davies D and Neal C, *Pink Therapy*. Oxford University Press, 1996.

Mason-John V (ed.), *Talking Black*. Cassell, 1995.
O'Connor N and Ryan J, *Wild Desires and Mistaken Identities*. Virago, 1993.

Black people/mental health

Fernando S, *Mental Health, Race and Culture*. Macmillan/MIND, 1991.
Fernando S (ed.), *Mental Health in a Multi-Ethnic Society*. Routledge, 1995.
Good Practice in Mental Health, *Not Just Black and White*, 1995.
Littlewood R and Lipsedge M, *Aliens and Alienists*. Routledge, 1989.
MIND, *AZ Race Issues in Mental Health*, 1996.
MIND's Policy on Black and Minority Ethnic People and Mental Health. MIND, 1993.
Wison M, *Mental Health and Britain's Black Communities*. King's Fund, 1993.

Ethics/values/practice

Adams R, *Self Help, Social Work and Empowerment*. Macmillan, 1990.
Barker P and Baldwin S, *Ethical Issues in Mental Health*. Chapman & Hall, 1991.
Banks S, *Ethics and Values in Social Work*. BASW/Macmillan, 1995.
Barham P and Hayward R, *Relocating Madness from the Mental Patient to the Person*. Free Association Books, 1995.
Dalley G, *Ideologies of Caring*, 2nd edn. BASW/Macmillan, 1996.
Dalrymple J and Burke B, *Anti-Oppressive Practice: Social Care and the Law*. Open University Press, 1995.
Dominelli L, *Anti-Racist Social Work*, 2nd edn. Macmillan, 1997.
Doyal L, Gough L, *A Theory of Human Need*. Macmillan, 1991.
Eagleton T, *The Illusions of Postmodernism*. Blackwell, 1996.
Friere P, *Pedagogy of Hope: Reliving Pedagogy of the Oppressed*. Continuum, 1996.
Hugman R and Smith D (eds), *Ethical Issues in Social Work*. Routledge, 1995.
Humphries B (ed.), *Critical Perspectives on Empowerment*. Venture Press, 1996.
Payne M, *Modern Social Work Theory*. Macmillan, 1991.
Prior L, *The Social Organisation of Mental Illness*. Sage, 1993.
Read J and Wallcraft J, *Guidelines on Advocacy for Mental Health Workers*. Unison/MIND, 1995.
Read J and Wallcraft J, *Guidelines on Equal Opportunities and Mental Health*. Unison/MIND, 1995.
Thompson N, *Anti-discriminatory Practice*. Macmillan, 1993.

Tronto JC, *Moral Boundaries: A Political Argument for an Ethics of Care.* Routledge, 1993.

Service user perspectives/general

Baker P, *The Voice Inside.* Hearing Voices Network, 1995.
Breggin P, *Toxic Psychiatry.* HarperCollins, 1993.
Diski J, *Monkey's Uncle.* Phoenix, 1994.
Hart L, *Phone at Nine Just To Say You're Alive.* Douglas Elliot, 1995.
Leader A, *Direct Power* (Resource Pack). CSN/BCS/MIND/Pavilion, 1995.
Lindow V, *Self-Help Alternatives to Mental Health Services.* MIND, 1994.
Millet K, *The Looney Bin Trip.* Virago, 1991.
Pembroke LR, *Self-Harm: Perspectives from Personal Experience.* Survivors Speak Out, 1994.
Read J and Reynolds J (eds), *Speaking our Minds: An Anthology.* Open University Press, 1996.
Rogers A, Pilgrim D and Lacey R, *Experiencing Psychiatry: User's Views of Services.* MIND/Macmillan, 1993.
Survivors Speak Out, *Under the Asylum Tree: Survivors Poetry*, 1995.
Thornton J (ed.), *Out of Mind: Out of Sight.* Yorkshire Art Circus, 1996.
Tudor K, *Mental Health Promotion.* Routledge, 1996.
Yalom ID, *Love's Executioner and Other Tales of Psychotherapy.* Penguin, 1989.

Community/health/support

Adams R, *Social Work and Empowerment.* BASW/Macmillan, 1996.
Brown A and Bourne I, *The Social Work Supervisor.* Open University Press, 1996.
Drew T and King M, *The Mental Health Handbook* (DK): *The complete guide to treatment, care and resources.* Piatkus, 1995.
Kelleher D and Hillier S, *Researching Cultural Differences in Health.* Routledge, 1996.
MIND, *Reshaping the Future: MIND's Model for Community Mental Health Care*, 1995.
Morgan S, *Community Mental Health.* Chapman & Hall, 1994.
Newton J, *Preventing Mental Illness in Practice.* Routledge, 1995.
Pilgrim D and Rogers A, *A Sociology of Mental Health and Illness.* Open University Press, 1993.
Pritchard J and Kemshall H, *Good Practice in Risk Assessment and Risk Management.* Jessica Kingsley Publishers, 1995.

Pritchard J, *Good Practice in Supervision: Statutory and Voluntary Organisations*. Good Practice Series. Jessica Kingsley, 1995.

Ramon S (ed.), *Beyond Community Care*. MIND/Macmillan, 1991.

Tomlinson D and Carrier J (eds), *Asylum in the Community*. Routledge, 1996.

Townsend P, Davidson N and Whitehead M, *Inequalities in Health: The Black Report/The Health Divide*. Penguin, 1992.

References

Adams L and Pintus P (1994) A challenge to prevailing theory and practice. *Critical Public Health* 5(2): 17–29.

Adams L (1996) In: Scriven A and Orme J (eds) *Health Promotion Professional Perspectives*. Buckingham: Open University Press.

Ahmad B (1990) *Black Perspectives in Social Work*. Birmingham: Venture Press.

Amies P (1996) Psychotherapy patients: are they the worried well? *Psychiatric Bulletin* 20: 153–156.

Anglia and Oxford Regional Health Authority (1994) *Making Sense of Purchasing: Looking to the Future*. Cambridge: A&ORHA.

Antonovsky A (1996) The salutogenic model as a theory to guide health promotion. *Health Promotion International* 11(1): 11–18.

Appleby L and Araya R (eds) (1991) *Mental Health Services in the Global Village*, Gaskell. London: Royal College of Psychiatrists.

Audit Commission (1994) *Finding a Place*. London: HMSO.

Austin W, Gallop R, Harris D and Spencer E (1996) A 'domains of practice' approach to the standards of psychiatric and mental health nursing. *Journal of Psychiatric and Mental Health Nursing* 3: 11–15.

Baldwin S and Priest R G (1995) Primary Care Psychiatry 1. Oxford: Rapid Communications. pp. 71–76.

Balogh R and Bond S (1995) Telling it like it is, Mental Health Audit. *Health Service Journal* March: 26–27.

Banks S (1995) *Ethics and Values in Social Work*. London: BASW/Macmillan.

Barham P and Hayward R (1995) *Relocating Madness: From the Mental Patient to the Person*. London: Free Association Books.

Barker P, Reynolds B, Whitehill I and Novak V (1996) Working with mental distress. *Nursing Times* 92(2): 25–27.

Barker P, Reynolds W and Stevenson C (1997) The human science basis of psychiatric nursing: theory and practice. *Journal of Advanced Nursing* 25: 660–667.

Barker P (1995) Promoting growth through community mental health nursing. *Mental Health Nursing* 15(3): 12–15.

Barnes M and Wistow G (1990) *Understanding User Involvement*. Leeds: Nuffield Institute Seminar Series.

Barnes M and Maple N (1992) *Women and Mental Health: Challenging the Stereotypes*. London: BASW/Ventura Press.

Bauman Z (1993) *Postmodern Ethics*. Oxford: Blackwell.

Benzeval M, Judge K and Whitehead M (eds) (1995) *Tacking Inequalities in Health: An Agenda for Action*. London: Kings Fund.

Beresford P (1990) *Researching Citizen-Involvement: A Collaborative or Colonising Enterprise? Open Services Project*. Leeds: Nuffield Institute Seminar Series.

Bewsher H (1995) *Tranx Self Help Initiatives*. Sheffield: Sheffield Health.

Black J (1992) *User Involvement in Mental Health Services: An Annotated Biography 1985–1992*. Birmingham: Department of Social Policy and Social Work, University of Birmingham.

Bostock J (1991) Developing a radical approach: the contribution and dangers of community psychology. *Clinical Psychology Forum* June 1991.

Boxer J and McCulloch G (1996) Mental health policy and practice. In: Gastrell P and Edwards J (eds) *Community Health Nursing: Frameworks for Practice.* London: Baillière Tindall.

Brager and Specht (1973) *Community Organising.* New York: Columbia University Press.

Braidwood E (1995) *Thinking Ahead: Mental Health Promotion Priorities and Planning.* Report by Hull and Holderness Community Health.

British Association of Psychopharmacology (1993) Guidelines for treating depressive illness with anti-depressants. *Journal of Psychopharmacology* 7(1): 19–23.

Brizer D (1993) *Psychiatry for Beginners.* London: Airlift Book Company.

Brochie J and Wann M (1993) *Training for Lay Participation in Health: Token Voices of the People?* London: The Patients Association.

Brooker C, Repper J and Booth A (1996) Examining effectiveness of community mental health nursing. *Mental Health Nursing* 16(3): 12–15.

Bury M, Gabe G and Wright Z (1994) *Promoting Mental Health: A Social Perspective – A Report for the Health Education Authority.* London: Department of Social Policy and Social Science, University of London.

Butcher H (1993) *Community and Public Policy.* Oxford: Pluto Press.

Butler T (1993) *Changing Mental Health Services: The Politics and Policy.* London: Chapman and Hall.

Butterworth T (1994) *Mental Health Nursing Review Team, Working in Partnership: A Collaborative Approach to Care.* London: Department of Health/HMSO.

The Calouste Gulbenkian Foundation (1968) *Community Work and Social Change in Current Issues in Community Work.* London: Routledge & Kegan Paul.

Campbell P (1995) *User Empowerment in Practice: The Joint Agenda.* Notes from a National Seminar on User Empowerment and Advocacy in Mental Health Services, May 1995, Manchester.

Caplan G (1961) *An Approach to Community Mental Health.* London: Tavistock.

Caplan R and Holland R (1990) Rethinking health education theory. *Health Education Journal* 49: 10–12.

Carabine J (1996) Empowering sexualities. In: Humphries B (ed.) *Critical Perspectives on Empowerment.* Birmingham: BASW/Venture Press.

The Children Act (1989). London: HMSO.

Clifford Beers Foundation (1996) *Enhanced Mental Health Promotion and Prevention in Europe: A Policy Paper.* Birmingham: University of Central England in Birmingham.

Cochrane R and Sashidharan S P (1996) Mental health and ethnic minorities: a review of literature and implications for services. In: *Ethnicity and Health: Reviews of Literature and Guidance for Purchasers in the Areas of Cardiovascular Disease, Mental Health and Haemoglobinopathies.* York: NHS Centre for Reviews and Dissemination, University of York.

Conlan E, Gell C, Graley R, Mooney I and Simpson T (1994) *Advocacy – A Code of Practice.* NHS Executive, Mental Health Task Force User Group.

Conway M, Melzer D, Shepard G and Troop P (1994) *A Companion to Purchasing Adult Mental Health Services.* Anglia and Oxford Regional Health Authority.

Cooper D (1971) *Introduction to Madness and Civilization Michel Foucault.* London: Routledge.

Cozens J and Firth CJF (1994) *Stress in Doctors: A Longitudinal Study. Research Commissioned by the Department of Health, Research & Development Initiative on Mental Health of the NHS Workforce.* Leeds: Department of Psychology, University of Leeds.

Craig G, Derricourt N and Loney M (eds) (1982) *Community Work and the State.* London: Routledge & Kegan Paul.

Dahlgren G and Whitehead M (1992) *Policies and Strategies to Promote Equality in Health*. Copenhagen: WHO.

Danneman H and Howland G (1996) Hey, trusts, can we climb on board? *IHSM Network* 3(9): 4–5.

Dalgard O S, Sorensen T and Bjork S (1991) Community psychiatry and health promotion research 18. In: Badura B and Kickbusch I (eds) *Health Promotion Research, Towards a New Social Epidemiology*. Geneva: WHO Regional Publications, 37.

Dalley G (1996) *Ideologies of Caring: Rethinking Community and Collectivism*, 2nd ed. London: Child Poverty Action Group/BASW/Macmillan.

Dalrymple J and Burke B (1995) *Anti-Oppressive Practice: Social Care and the Law*. Buckingham: Open University Press.

Deacon M and Dark P (1994) *Promoting Mental Health Through Purchasing: Conference Report and Checklist for Developing a Mental Health Promotion Specification*. South Thames Regional Health Authority.

Department of Health (1989a) *Caring for People: Community Care in the Next Decade and Beyond*. London: HMSO.

Department of Health (1989b) *Working for Patients, Cmnd. 555*. London: HMSO.

Department of Health (1990) *National Health Service and Community Care Act*. London: HMSO.

Department of Health (1991) *The Patients' Charter (E1 (91) 128)*. London: HMSO.

Department of Health (1992a) *The Health of the Nation: A Strategy for Health in England*. London: HMSO.

Department of Health (1992b) *Local Voices: The Views of Local People in Purchasing for Health*. London: NHS Management Executive.

Department of Health (1993a) *The Health of the Nation – Key Area Handbook: Mental Illness*. London: HMSO.

Department of Health (1993b) *Nursing in Primary Health Care: New World, New Opportunities*. London: NHS Management Executive.

Department of Health (1993c) *Working Together for Better Health*. London: HMSO.

Department of Health (1994a) *The Health of the Nation – Key Area Handbook: Mental Illness*, 2nd edn. London: HMSO.

Department of Health (1994b) *Targeting Practice: The Contribution of Nurses, Midwives and Health Visitors to The Health of the Nation*. London: HMSO.

Department of Health (1995a) *Together We Stand: Child and Adolescent Mental Health Services – NHS Health Advisory Service*. London: HMSO.

Department of Health (1995b) *Making it Happen – Public Health: The Contribution, Role and Development of Nurses, Midwives and Health Visitors*. Report of the Standing Nursing and Midwifery Advisory Committee (SNMAC).

Department of Health (1995c) *Variations in Health: What can the Department of Health and the NHS do?* London: HMSO.

Department of Health (1995d) *Fit for the Future, Second Progress Report on the Health of the Nation*. London: HMSO.

Department of Health (1995e) *Building Bridges: A Guide to arrangements for Inter-Agency Working for the Care and Protection of Severely Mentally Ill People*. London: HMSO.

Department of Health (1995f) *The Health of the Nation – ABC of Mental Health in the Workplace: A Resource Pack for Employers*. London: HMSO.

Department of Health (1996a) *Primary Care: The Future*. London: NHS Executive.

Department of Health (1996b) *Mental Health at Work: Health of the Nation at Work*. London: HMSO.

Department of Health (1996c) *Spectrum of Care*. London: HMSO.

Dominelli L (1997a) *Sociology for Social Work*. London: Macmillan.

Dominelli L (1997b) *Anti-Racist Social Work*, 2nd ed. London: BASW/Macmillan.

Dominelli L and McLeod E (1992) *Feminist Social Work*. London: Macmillan.

Donaldson L (1995) The Listening Blank. *Health Service Journal* 21 September.

Downie R S, Fyfe C and Tannahill A (1990) *Health Promotion Models and Values*. Oxford: Oxford University Press.

Duggan M (1995) *Primary Health Care: A Prognosis.* London: Institute for Public Policy Research.

Elliott A (1992) *Social Theory and Psychoanalysis in Transition: Self and Society from Freud to Kristeva.* Oxford: Blackwell.

Eskin F (1992) Daydream believers. *Health Service Journal* September 10. p.24.

Faculty of Public Health Medicine (1996) *Towards Commissioning Quality District Services.* London: Faculty of Public Health Medicine.

Fernando S (1993) Mental Health for All. In: Beattie and Gott (eds) *Health and Wellbeing: A Reader.* Buckingham: Open University Press.

Fernando S (1991) *Mental Health, Race and Culture.* Basingstoke: Macmillan Press.

Friere P (1996) *Pedagogy of Hope: Reliving Pedagogy of the Oppressed.* New York: Continuum Publishing.

Funnell R, Oldfield K and Speller V (1995) *Towards Healthier Alliances.* London: HEA.

Gates B (1995) Whose Best Interest? *Nursing Times,* January, 31–32.

Giddens A (1993) *Sociology,* 2nd edn. Oxford: Polity.

Gillon R (1985) *Philosophical Medical Ethics.* Chichester: John Wiley & Sons.

Glasman D (1991) The challenge of patient power. *Health Service Journal,* September: 16–17.

Goodstadt MS, Simpson RI, Loranger PL (1987) Health promotion: a conceptual integration. *American Journal of Health Promotion* 1(3): 58–63.

Green J (1992) *Mediawise* 7, Spring Mental Health Media Quarterly. London: Mental Health Media.

Green M, Martin M and Williams J (1996) Critical Consciousness or Commercial Consciousness? Dilemmas in Higher Education. In: Humphries B (ed.) *Critical Perspectives on Empowerment.* Birmingham: BASW/Venture Press.

Greenoak J, Letherbridge J and Hunt R (1994) *Mental Health Priorities for Action. Executive Summary.* HEA internal document.

Ham C (1992) *Health Policy in Britain: The Politics and Organisation of the National Health Service,* 3rd ed. London: Macmillan.

Hamlin C (1996) The real challenge for the new authorities. *IHSM Network* 3 (5): p.1.

Harrison K (1996) *Horrible Hybrids.* London: Open Mind.

Health Education Authority Mental Health Factsheet (1996) *Mental Health Promotion – Issues for Black and Minority Ethnic People.* London: Health Education Authority.

Health Gain Investment Programme Technical Review Document (1994) *People with Mental Health Problems (Part One).* London: The Centre for Mental Health Services Development, Kings College.

Healthy Sheffield (1991) *Our City – Our Health: Ideas for Improving Health in Sheffield.* Sheffield: Sheffield Development Unit.

Healthy Sheffield (1993) *Community Development and Health: The Way Forward in Sheffield.* Sheffield: Sheffield Development Unit.

Hoggert P and Hambleton R (1987) *Decentralisation and Democracy: Localising Public Services.* Bristol: School of Advanced Urban Studies, University of Bristol.

Holland S (1992) From social abuse to social action: a neighbourhood psychotherapy and social action project for women. *Changes* 16: 146–153.

Hornby S (1993) *Collaborative Care: Interprofessional, Interagency, and Interpersonal.* Oxford: Blackwell.

Hosman C and Veltman N (1994) *Prevention in Mental Health: A Review of the Effectiveness of Health Education and Health Promotion.* Geneva: WHO.

Hugman R and Smith D (eds) (1995) *Ethical Issues in Social Work.* London: Routledge.

Humphries B (1996) *Critical Perspectives on Empowerment*. Birmingham: BASW/Venture Press.

Hunter D J and Harrison S (1993) *Effective Purchasing for Health Care: Proposals for the First Five Years, A Report for the NHS Management Executive*. Leeds: Nuffield Institute for Health.

Jones A (1996) The value of Peplau's theory for mental health nursing. *British Journal of Nursing* 5(14): 877–881.

Jones K (1994) *The Making of Social Policy in Britain 1830–1990*, 2nd edn. London: The Athlone Press.

Kavanagh K H and Kennedy P H (1992) *Promoting Cultural Diversity*. London: Sage.

Kelleher C (1996) Education and training in health promotion: theory and methods. *Health Promotion International* 11(1): 47–53.

Kopp S (1974) *If You Meet the Buddha on the Road, Kill Him!* London: Sheldon Press.

Lago C and Thompson J (1996) *Race, Culture and Counselling*. Buckingham: Open University Press.

Leader A (1995) *Direct Power: A Resource Pack for People Who Want to Develop Their Own Care Plans and Support Networks*. London: Pavilion Publishing/MIND.

Leeds Declaration. In: Eskin F (1994) The Leeds Declaration: refocusing public health research for action. *Critical Public Health* 5(3): 39–44.

Leonard J (1994) *Interacting: Multimedia and Health*. London: Health Education Authority.

Lemma A (1996) *Introduction to Psychopathology*. London: Sage.

Lewis J and Glennerster H (1996) *Implementing The New Community Care*. Buckingham: Open University Press.

Lindow V (1991) Towards user power. *Health Service Journal* August 18.

Lindow V (1996) What we want from community psychiatric nurses. In Read J and Reynolds J (eds) *Speaking Our Minds: An Anthology*. Buckingham: Open University Press.

Lynn E and Muir A (1996) Empowerment in social work: the case of CCETSW's Welsh language policy. In: Humphries B (ed.) *Critical Perspectives on Empowerment*. Birmingham: BASW/Venture Press.

MacDonald G (1994) *Promoting Mental Health: A Report for the Health Education Department*.

MacDonald J J and Warren W G (1991) Primary health care as an educational process: a model and a Freirean perspective. *Community Health Education* 12(1): 35–50.

MacDonald S (1991) *An Equal Under the Act: A Practice Guide to the Children's Act*.

Magowan R (1994) *Purchasing for MHP – A Potential Shopping List for Consideration, Discussion and Refinement*. Sheffield: Trent RHA.

Malby B (ed.) (1995) *Clinical Audit for Nurses and Therapists*. London: Scutari Press.

Mallinson (1995) The social care task: social care association. In: Dalrymple J and Burke B (eds) *Anti-Oppressive Practice: Social Care and the Law*. Buckingham: Open University Press.

Mandela N (1994) *Long Walk to Freedom*. London: Little, Brown & Company.

McCormick K (1993) *Speaking out for the Public's Health, Papers from a Conference on Public Health Advocacy*. Birmingham: The Public Health Alliance.

McIver S and Martin G (1996) Guidelines on involving users in developing local patients' charters. *Patient's Charter News* December 1995.

Medical Campaign Project (1990) *Understanding Health Services: A Guide to the Recent Changes in the Organization of Health Services for Voluntary Organizations*. London: Medical Campaign Project.

Mensah J (1996) Everybody's problem. *Nursing Times* 92 (22): 26–27.

The Mental Health Act Commission (1993–1995) *Sixth Biennial Report*. London: HMSO.

Mental Health Foundation (1994) *Creating Community Care. Inquiry into Community Care for People with Severe Mental Illness*. London: Mental Health Foundation.

MIND (1994a) *Policy 1, The Health of the Nation, Involving Users in the National Targets*. London: MIND Publications.

MIND (1994b) *The Right to Know*. London: MIND Publications.

MIND (1994c) *The Breakthrough Campaign*. London: MIND Publications.

MIND (1995) *Reshaping the Future: MIND's Model for Community Mental Health Care 1-874690-29-4*. London: MIND Publications.

Mohammed S (1993) *User Sensitive Purchasing*. London: Kings Fund.

Moodley P (1993) Setting up services for ethnic minorities. In: Bhugra D and Leff J (eds) (1993) *Principles of Social Psychiatry*. Oxford: Blackwell.

Monach J and Spriggs L (1995) *Mental Health Promotion in Sheffield*. Sheffield: Department of Psychiatry, University of Sheffield/Sheffield Hallam University.

Money MC (1996) Mental health not mental illness: a positive community approach. *The Journal of Contemporary Health*: 56–58.

Morrall P (1996) Clinical sociology and the empowerment of clients. *Mental Health Nursing* 16(3): 24–27.

Naidoo J and Wills J (1994) *Health Promotion: Foundations for Practice*. London: Baillière Tindall.

Newton J (1988) *Preventing Mental Illness*. London: Routledge.

Newton J (1992) *Preventing Mental Illness in Practice*. London: Routledge.

NHS Directorate (1993) *Protocol for Investment in Health Gain, Mental Health*. Welsh Office: Welsh Health Planning Forum.

NHS Executive (1994a) *Building on Experience: A Training Pack for Mental Health Service Users Working as Trainers, Speakers and Workshop Facilitators*. Task Force User Group. Weatherby: DOH.

NHS Executive (1994b) *Guidelines for a Local Charter for Users of Mental Health Services*. Weatherby: DOH.

NHS Executive (1995) *Priorities and Planning Guidance for the NHS 1996–97*. Leeds: NHS Executive.

NHS Executive Trent (1994a) *Focus on User Empowerment in Mental Health Care: An Aid to Contracting*.

NHS Executive Trent (1994b) *Purchasing Health Services for Men East Midlands Men's Health Network*.

NHSME (1992) *Making Local Voices Heard in Purchasing or Health Annex A (16)*.

NHSME (1993) *Purchasing for Health: A framework for action. The Vision for Purchasing*. A speech by Dr B Mawhinney at the Association for Public Health, 29th April 1993.

North N (1995) Fundholding and commissioning in 2000 – Goliath, David or just history? *Critical Public Health* 6(1): 11–19.

North Western Mental Health Promotion Group (1994) *Health of the Nation Targets for Mental Illness: The Contribution of Preventative Approaches*. A report from the East Lancashire Health Consortium.

Nuffield Institute (1993) Depression in primary care. *Effective Health Care Bulletin* 5.

Ong B N (1993) *The Practice for Health Services Research*. London: Chapman & Hall.

Oxford Modern English Dictionary (1993). Oxford: Oxford University Press.

Payne M (1991) *Modern Social Work Theory: A Critical Introduction*. London: Macmillan.

Patel N (1995) In search of the Holy Grail. In: Hugman R and Smith D (eds) *Ethical Issues in Social Work*. London: Routledge.

Pearson G (1975) *The Deviant Imagination: Psychiatry, Social Work and Social Change.* London: Macmillan.

Peckham S (1996) NHS policy developments. In: Gastrell P and Edwards J (eds) *Community Health Nursing.* London: Baillière Tindall.

Phillipson (1992). In: Dalrymple J and Burke B (eds) *Anti-Oppressive Practice: Social Care and the Law.* Buckingham: Open University Press.

Philo P, Henderson L and McLaughlin G (1992) *Mass Media Representations of Mental Health/Illness.* Scotland: Report for Health Education Board.

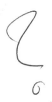

Pilgrim D (1993) Mental health services in the twenty-first century: the user-professional divide? In: Bornat J, Pereira C, Pilgrim D and Williams F (eds) *Community Care: A Reader.* London: Macmillan.

Prior L (1993) *The Social Organization of Mental Illness.* London: Sage Publications.

Pritchard P (1993) *Partnerships with Patients: A Practice Guide to Starting a Patient Participation Group,* 3rd edn. London: The Royal College of General Practitioners.

Quinn J B (1992) The strategy concept. In: Mintzberg H and Quinn J B (eds) *The Strategy Process: Concepts and Contexts.* New Jersey: Prentice Hall.

Ranade W (1994) *A Future for the NHS? Health Care in the 1990s.* London: Longman.

Read J and Reynolds J (eds) (1996) *Speaking our Minds: An Anthology.* Buckingham: Open University Press.

Read J and Wallcraft J (1995) *Guidelines on Equal Opportunities and Mental Health.* London: MIND Publications.

Rigge M (1995) Does public opinion matter? *Health Service Journal* 7th September.

Rogers A, Pilgrim D and Lacey R (1993) *Experiencing Psychiatry: Users' Views of Services.* London: MIND Publications.

Rogers A and Pilgrim D (1996) *Mental Health Policy in Britain, A Critical Introduction.* London: Macmillan.

Ross D, Campbell P and Neeter R (1993) Community care: users' perspectives. In: Barnham P (ed.) *Closing the Asylum, The Mental Patient in Modern Society.* London: Penguin.

Ross K (1995) Speaking in tongues: involving users in day care services. *British Journal of Social Work,* 25(6).

Royal College of Nursing (RCN) (1993) *The Role of Nurses in Purchasing for Health Gain.* London: RCN.

Rudman M J (1996) User involvement in the nursing curriculum: seeking user's views *Journal of Psychiatric and Mental Health Nursing* 3: 195–200.

Sang B (1994) The user as commissioner. *Kings Fund News,* 17(4).

Sartorious N (1996) quoted in conference papers: *Setting the New Agenda; Effective Skills in Mental Health Promotion,* 1996. Birmingham: The Clifford Beers Foundation, University of Central England in Birmingham.

Sedgwick P (1983) *Psycho Politics.* London: Pluto Press.

Sheffield Health Promotion (1996) *Policy Paper on Health Promotion.* Sheffield: Sheffield Health.

Sheffield Mental Health Promotion Group (1992) Sheffield Health.

Sheffield Strategy For Adult Mental Health (1996) *Sheffield Health, Family and Community Services.* Sheffield: Community Health Sheffield NHS Trust.

Sivanandan A (1993) The Black Politics of Health. *Race and Class* 34(4).

Smithies J, Adams L, Webster G and Beattie A (1990) *Community Participation in Health Promotion.* London: Health Education Authority.

Snell P (1994) *Framework for Action, Healthy Sheffield Report.* Sheffield: Healthy Sheffield.

Spinelli E (1994) *Demystifying Therapy.* London: Constable.

Stark W (1986) The politics of primary prevention in mental health: the need for a theoretical basis. *Health Promotion* 1(2): 179–185.

Stoddard M (ed.) (1993) *The Sayings of Friedrich Nietzsche*. London: Duckworth.

Tannahill A (1985) What is health promotion? *Health Education Journal*, 44(4): 167–168.

Thompson A and Mathias P (1994) *Mental Health and Disorder*. London: Baillière Tindall.

Thompson N (1993) *Anti-Discriminatory Practice*. London: Macmillan.

Thompson N (1995). In: Dalrymple J and Burke B (eds) *Anti-Oppressive Practice: Social Care and the Law*. Buckingham: Open University Press.

Tilford S (1995) Mental health education – some issues. *Health Education and Research* 20(4): i–vii.

Tones K and Tilford S (1994) *Health Education, Effectiveness, Efficiency and Equity*, 2nd edn. London: Chapman and Hall.

Trent Regional Health Authority (1994) *Focus on Promoting Mental Health at Work in the NHS: An Aid to Contracting*. Sheffield: Trent Regional Health Authority.

Tronto J C (1993) *Moral Boundaries: A Political Argument for an Ethics of Care*. London: Routledge.

Tudor K (1996) *Mental Health Promotion*. London: Routledge.

UNCED (1992) *Agenda 21* (United Nations Conference on Environment and Development).

Wallace R (1993) Social Disintegration and the Spread of AIDS – II: Meltdown of Sociogeographic Structure in Urban Minority Neighbourhood. *Social Science and Medicine* 37: 887–896.

Whitehead M (1990) *The Concepts and Principles of Equity and Health*. Copenhagen: WHO Regional Office for Europe.

Whitehead M (1995) Tackling inequalities: a review of policy initiatives. In: Benzeval M, Judge K and Whitehead M (eds) *Tackling Inequalities of Health: An Agenda for Action*. London: Kings Fund.

WHO (1978) *The Declaration at Alma Ata: Health for All, series 1*. Geneva: WHO.

WHO (1986) *Ottowa Charter: The First International Conference on Health Promotion, 21 November 1986*. Geneva: WHO.

WHO (1991) *Health for All Targets: European Health for All Series No 4*. The Health Policy for Europe. Geneva: WHO.

WHO (1994) *Action for Health in Cities*. Copenhagen: WHO Regional Office for Europe.

Williams J, Watson G, Smith H, Copperman J and Wood D (1993) *Purchasing Effective Mental Health Services for Women: A Framework for Action*. London: MIND Publications.

Williams R and Morgan H G (eds) (1994) *Suicide Prevention July, 1994, The Challenge Confronted, HAS*. London: HMSO.

Wilson J (1995) *Two Worlds: Self help groups and professionals*. Birmingham: British Association of Social Workers.

Wycherley B (1987) In: Farrell E (ed.) *Living Skills, Life Matters*. Conference Report, South East Thames Regional Health Authority.

Yalom I D (1980) *Existential Psychotherapy*. London: Basic Books.

Index